PRAISE FOR

"Lentz's Accidental Journey is much more than another book outlining recovery from a severe traumatic brain injury (TBI). It is a novel that describes the effect on the survivor and the heartbreak of the family in the aftermath of a devastating injury. The survivor becomes like an alien self to his family, present and not present, with damaged self-awareness and unmistakable consequences. This book is a complex tapestry of hope, mingled with despair, and a solution that saves an otherwise broken marriage."

–John W. Cassidy, MD, Co-Founder of the Neuropsychiatry TBI Program at McLean Hospital, Boston, and Founder and CEO of Nexus Health Systems, Houston

"Richard Lentz has written a novel abounding with life's complications. At once a probing family saga and the story of a man's recovery from a traumatic brain injury, *Accidental Journey* is the richest sort of book. It immerses you in the injury, then pulls you out on the other side. You'll feel as if you've gone through the recovery yourself, and, standing at the crossroads you find on the light end of the tunnel, you'll be as resolute as these finely drawn characters. You'll also be wiser. And fuller of heart."

–Peter Geye, author of *The Ski Jumpers*

"Dr. Lentz carefully informed his narrative by drawing from not only relevant science on brain injury, but also through a several year process of consultation with clinicians who treat brain injuries in a rehabilitation setting. With this, in addition to his own rich clinical experience, he gives a novel that treats the experience of brain injury with both wisdom and compassion, recognizing the many factors that shape recovery and adaptation.

–Kyle Harvison, PhD, ABPP, Board Certified Clinical Neuropsychologist

"An important book that chronicles the emotional journey faced by a family in the wake of a traumatic brain injury. *Accidental Journey* is filled with insights about marriage, love, and commitment as Jeff and Cate navigate the uncertain future after a life-altering accident. Leading the reader into the inner worlds of its characters as well as the medical complexity of a traumatic brain injury, *Accidental Journey* shows us what it means to be human in an imperfect and uncertain world. Richard Lentz, M.D., has crafted a powerful work of fiction that captures with honesty and compassion the transformations of a family in the aftermath of traumatic injury."

–Leslie Morris, Beverly and Richard Professor in Liberal Arts, Professor of German, University of Minnesota, Co-convenor of research collaborative on Narrative Medicine, Institute for Advanced Study, University of Minnesota

"Although each brain injury recovery is unique, there are common hurdles and challenges that unite this community of survivors, family members and loved ones. Richard Lentz does a remarkable job of weaving these issues together and strikes the perfect balance of humor and heartbreak in telling the tale of one family's journey."

–David King, Chief Executive Officer, Minnesota Brain Injury Alliance

"*Accidental Journey* is a well-researched novel based on the realities of life after successful Jeff suffers a traumatic brain injury in a car accident, causing impairment of memory, emotional responses, and cognition with devastating effects on job performance, marriage, parenting, friendships, and coping with daily events. Dr. Lentz does a masterful job describing the effects on Jeff, Cate and the children. Although this account is fictitious, readers who have experienced the familial effects of serial concussions or significant brain injuries will find recognizable situations and insights."

–Jennine Speier, MD, Physiatrist and Retired Director of Courage Kenny Rehabilitation Institute, Allina Health System, Minneapolis

"Richard Lentz has created an astute psychological portrait of a woman caught between her own needs and a necessary recalibration of her marriage. Her paradoxical solution turns conventional morality on its head–a thought-provoking read."

–Gloria A. Levin, PsyD, LP, Psychoanalyst/therapist

"Love isn't simple. *Accidental Journey* makes that clear, as Lentz deftly weaves a woman's quest for love with the story of her husband's traumatic brain injury—a quest that leads her to the realization that her only way to happiness is to lead a double life."

–Brian Duren, award-winning author of *Whiteout*

"*Accidental Journey* should be required reading for any individual or family member who has experienced traumatic brain injury. And for the rest of us who are just curious, Richard Lentz does a masterful job explaining the consequences of a devastating brain injury. He shows the reader how it changes a person, a marriage, a family, and every aspect of lives that must endure. *Accidental Journey* is worth the read."

–Cary Griffith, author of the novel, *Cougar Claw*, and winner of the Minnesota Book Award for Nonfiction

"Two collisions catapult the reader into this debut novel, setting in motion a family's intimate encounter with love, loss, and an ambiguous future. First, Jeff and Cate, married with two young children and successful careers, having made a virtue out of avoidance, vigorously confront each other, raising hope for a better future. Then, a head-on collision leaves Jeff battling a traumatic brain injury, fighting to restore as much of himself as possible, and leaving his family in shatters. With great sensitivity, Lentz describes the impact of these two collisions in a book that is well paced, painfully slow and paradoxically urgent. A must read for any family that has experienced traumatic brain injury, or for any reader interested in the dynamic interplay of heart and medical science."

–Hal Steiger, PhD, LP, Psychoanalyst

"Accidental Journey is a riveting account of a family upended by traumatic brain injury. We learn along with Cate what it means to be married to someone whose brain has been 'busted' by a head-on car collision. Cate is a survivor, and so is her husband Jeff, but he is now a different version of himself. As Cate and their children Kayla and Ben struggle to adjust to their new reality, we are introduced to the basic facts of TBI from an expert in the field. Psychiatrist Richard Lentz offers a compelling, compassionate, and scientifically accurate account of this complex condition—and (just as importantly) how to cope with it.

–Madelon Sprengnether, author of *Crying at the Movies*, and *Mourning Freud*.

Accidental Journey

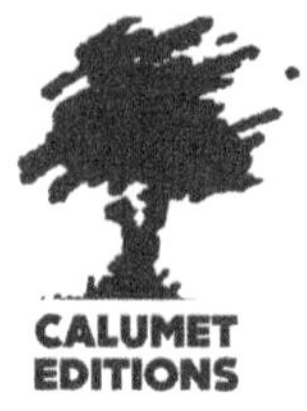

Minneapolis

Second Edition December 2022

10 9 8 7 6 5 4 3 2

ISBN: 978-1-959770-18-3

Cover and book design by Gary Lindberg

Accidental Journey

Richard D. Lentz

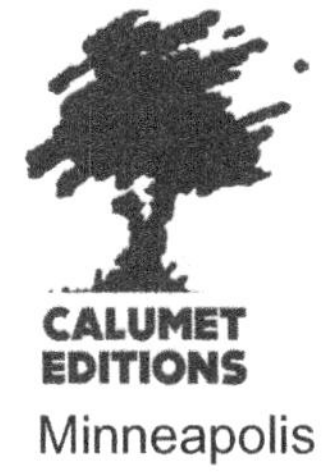

Minneapolis

To Joanie for her constant support, and to Daniel and Andrew.
And to all those individuals and families who suffer from traumatic brain injury

CHAPTER ONE:

The Day before Thanksgiving, 2012

Cate entered the grounds of the Como Park Zoo and Conservatory in St. Paul a few steps ahead of Jeff and her two children. She hoped to arrange a private conversation with Meg for later that afternoon or perhaps tomorrow after their families shared Thanksgiving dinner.

Last evening, Jeff had suggested a family day at the zoo, just the four of them. But Cate wanted to invite friends rather than be alone with Jeff, even with the kids as a buffer. She knew it wasn't fair to blame everything on him—she contributed to the chasm that had opened between them—yet she felt hurt and angry and surmised that Jeff did too. In the past year, he'd stopped listening to her and became disinterested and, at times, remote. And she'd stopped listening to him.

It hadn't always been that way. For most of the past twelve years, she and Jeff would build a fire and sit on the family room couch, holding hands, talking about their children, nurturing each other's demanding careers, but lately, they'd begun to sit on separate chairs.

Cate and the children—ten-year-old Kayla and eight-year-old Ben—loved zoos, and Jeff knew it; his suggestion was vintage Jeff. As a child in St. Louis, Cate had dragged her family to the zoo so often that her parents offered to let her live there in her own cage. Cate read animal bedtime stories to Kayla and Ben, who adored them.

"Why not just us?" Jeff asked when Cate insisted they'd have more fun if Meg's family joined them. "You always say zoos are for families."

"We'll have two families, and I can finalize Thanksgiving plans with Meg," said Cate. Meg and Scott's kids, Evie and David, were the same ages as Kayla and Ben. The two girls and two boys were best friends, and the dads and the moms were close.

Jeff offered a rueful smile. "You know it's not the same."

"The zoo was a lovely idea, and we'll have fun."

"Okay, if you agree to make time this weekend, Cate. You and I need to talk."

"Fine. We'll talk."

* * *

At the zoo, fresh clouds permeated the fall sky, thick enough to keep ground warmth from escaping after three warmer-than-usual days, porous enough to dapple the zoo with sunlight.

Kayla and Ben spied their friends and ran toward them, shouting. Cate spotted Meg and waved. The men grinned, and the families headed for the seal exhibit, where Jeff and Scott handed the boys money to buy buckets of fish to feed them; the girls declined the offer of "icky" fish. The moms found benches alongside the tanks and sat watching the boys feed the seals and the girls bury their faces in smartphones.

"Tweens grow smartphones along with breasts," said Meg.

"Yup. Jeff was more prepared for that than I was," said Cate.

"The phone or the breasts?"

"Probably both." Cate laughed. They chatted about shopping for training bras with the girls, agreeing that pubertal girls were fun for moms, joking that puberty for boys meant deodorant and smelly socks. "I'll let Jeff handle the deodorant," said Cate.

"And leave you with the smelly socks?" asked Meg. Cate looked at Jeff and couldn't keep tears from her eyes. "Cate," said Meg, "what's going on?"

"It's bad. I was hoping we could get together later, just us?" They settled on a walk around Lake of the Isles in south Minneapolis later that afternoon for a heart-to-heart and to savor the last breath of fall. The forecast warned of a blizzard and a fifty-degree drop in temperature.

The earth smelled of decaying leaves on this warm fall day after a midnight rain. Cate spotted a dead fish on the ground, grabbed it with a sheet of newspaper that someone had left on the bench, and tossed it to the seals.

"Mom, we're going to see the giraffes," said Ben. He scurried toward the giraffe pen as his friend David and the dads followed, Kayla and Evie lagging behind, chatting and laughing.

Cate and Meg waved and stayed seated. They'd been close friends since their freshman year of college and could read each other's minds. "I knew there were problems, but not like this," said Meg.

Cate dabbed at her eyes and managed a wry smile. "This isn't the best time. Right now, it's easier to talk about zoos."

"Okay," said Meg. "Zoos. Let's see; you dragged me to my first zoo in Philadelphia when we were freshmen at Penn and to my second zoo when I visited you in St. Louis during spring too. How am I doing?"

"You're distracting me. Keep going."

"The St. Louis Zoo was my favorite," said Meg. "If we take our families to see it, you can make believe the trip is for the kids, like those bedtime animal stories you read to yourself and pretend are for them."

"Come on; they love those stories."

"So do you."

When Cate and Meg reached the giraffe pen, Ben was spewing giraffe facts. "Bet you don't know that he gets most of his water from food and goes weeks without drinking. If he needs water from the ground, he kneels or spreads his front legs." Ben loved giraffes. Mazy, named for maze-like reticulations, guarded one corner of his bedroom. His favorite book was *Zarafa*, a story about a Masai giraffe who sailed from Africa to Marseille with a hole cut in the hold for her head, then walked five hundred miles to Paris.

"Awesome. He's full of information, just like Jeff," said Meg.

"I like that he knows a lot, but I worry he's pedantic," said Cate softly.

Meg raised her eyebrows. Ben described the giraffe's face, the big eyes with prominent lashes, leaf-shaped ears, tiny horns, and jaws that chewed side to side like a camel. Everyone looked up and smiled.

"He sounds like a bright kid who loves giraffes," said Meg.

"I know. At this age, it's adorable," said Cate.

After the giraffes, they trudged to the zoo's restaurant for hot dogs and burgers, then to the adjacent conservatory to see the fall flower show. While the men talked, the girls hung out with cellphones, and the boys ran among ornamental grasses, Cate and Meg sat out of earshot in a hidden corner, surrounded by red and white chrysanthemums. "We're alone for the moment. Do you want to say more?"

"It's hard to say what I'm thinking."

"Maybe you should have kept Scott when you had him and not introduced him to me." Cate and Scott, Meg's husband, had dated before Cate met Jeff.

"No, I did the right thing because you and Scott were meant for each other. I used to think Jeff and I were too. Lately, I've been thinking you got the better deal."

"A year ago, you wouldn't have said that," said Meg. "No one goes from all good to all bad in a year. He loves you and the kids, and you both love your family."

"Thing is, I don't know if I want this marriage."

"Wow," said Meg. "That's huge."

Cate choked back tears.

"I'm shocked. You always dreamed of a personal life that was calm and secure." Meg gripped Cate's arm as they heard footsteps and saw the others approach. Cate put on her mom smile. The children wanted to see the lions before they left.

"What did you talk about? Love and marriage?" said Scott.

Jeff laughed.

"Just marriage," said Meg, with a quick glance at Cate.

* * *

Six weeks earlier, Cate had planned a Sunday excursion with Jeff and the kids to the Minnesota Landscape Arboretum, a place they all loved, hoping that an excursion to see fall colors would rekindle the fun in their lives. They started with brunch in the café.

"Spring sap makes fall syrup," said Jeff, as Kayla and Ben poured maple syrup onto waffles. He showed them iPhone pictures from their last visit, when sap from tapped maples flowed into buckets and bags, and Kayla and Ben stood laughing in front of the Sugarhouse evaporator.

In other pictures from the spring visit, the Arboretum glistened with early blossoms—snowdrops in the Hosta Glade, pussy willow buds on Green Heron Pond, and forsythia that didn't always bloom in Minnesota. Cate, a former gymnast and current marathoner, looked trim and cute in jeans and a white blouse with a sandy brown cardigan that matched the highlights in her dark brown hair. Jeff looked handsome in a University of Minnesota hoodie, maroon and gold, and khaki pants, still tanned from winter skiing.

But even last spring, Cate and Jeff had begun to stand apart.

Cate looked up from the pictures and studied Jeff as they munched on their October breakfast. Although he smiled at the kids, tension creased his eyes. She put her hand on his and caressed it. He turned his hand over and squeezed hers. Cate looked again at the pictures, at the happy kids.

"You guys have grown a lot in the past seven months," said Cate. Ben had become a Jeff doppelgänger, a square-faced miniature with bushy eyebrows, electric blue eyes, and light brown hair, his frame more elongated and muscled. Kayla, with Cate's soft brown eyes and Jeff's full lips, had become more like a woman, a few inches taller, her waist thinner, her dark brown hair longer and carefully brushed.

After brunch, they piled into the car to enjoy the fall foliage on the three-mile Arboretum drive. Autumnal colors, red and orange maples with stubborn leaves of green, hugged the trunks and lingered on lower branches; there were yellow bursts of aspen and birch and oaks fading into muted maroon.

Jeff parked the car, and they walked along the hiking trail, where pockets of goldenrod and purple spikes of blazing star had not yet faced a killing frost. Signs identified yellow sunflowers, violet asters, Russian sage, Celosia, eyeball plants, and sedum. They found the display of cucurbits—pumpkins, squash, and gourds—and beautiful scarecrow arrangements that pleased Cate and Jeff as much as the children, reminding Cate of her first visit with Jeff to the Arboretum in the fall of 2001, four and a half months before Kayla arrived. Cate kissed Jeff's cheek. He smiled and put his arm around her.

On the way home, Cate sat as close to Jeff as bucket seats would allow and put a hand on his thigh.

"Hey, Dad, can we stop at McDonald's?" asked Ben. Jeff drove without answering, and Cate felt herself bristle. Ben tapped his dad's shoulder twice, then twice again, a gesture Cate recognized as anxiety. "Can't we stop, Dad?" Jeff still didn't answer. Ben two-tapped again.

"For heaven's sake, Jeff, answer your son," said Cate.

"Huh?" said Jeff.

"I want to go to McDonald's, Dad," said Ben, exasperated.

"I'm hungry too," said Kayla.

"Okay, we can stop," said Jeff.

"No, we can't," said Cate, in her mom voice, to Jeff. "Can't you remember anything? The kids wanted tuna fish salad for lunch, and I made their favorite recipe." She shifted away from Jeff, toward the door.

"They want McDonald's. We can have tuna salad for dinner."

"You said you'd grill burgers for dinner. That's what I planned." She looked out the window at fall sumac, still red and beautiful. Her irritation disturbed her; she was usually affable. She turned to Jeff and softened her tone. "Honey, let's do what we decided. Besides, tuna is healthier than McDonald's."

"Okay," Jeff said. But his face had grown tight.

When they reached home, Jeff kindled a fire and picked up the newspaper. Usually, they worked together in the kitchen. Ben set the table and Kayla helped Cate assemble the sandwiches. From the door to the family room, Cate studied Jeff and felt sadness and disappointment.

CHAPTER TWO:

Afternoon

Cate and Meg talked first about Thanksgiving plans as they drove toward Lake of the Isles. Almost everything was ready for the feast, a brined turkey that Cate would stuff and put in the oven, garlic green beans for the stove, a sweet potato casserole, a pecan pie that Jeff would smoke on the grill, and a cranberry mold, roasted vegetables, and creamy mashed potatoes contributed by Meg. Jeff's parents would come early to help; Karen would bring pumpkin pie and Dan would teach Jeff how to make his famous corn pudding, passing down a family tradition.

Cate grimaced when Meg mentioned Dan.

"I thought you liked Jeff's dad," said Meg.

"I like him a lot. He's funny, smart, and a good guy, but sometimes he doesn't listen, like Jeff. Lately, that bugs me."

"You and Karen have the same problem. Have you talked with her?"

"A little. Mostly, she lives with it." Cate's face reddened, and she stepped up the pace.

They reached Lake of the Isles, one of a chain of lakes in the heart of Minneapolis surrounded by parkland, exited the car, and started to circle the lake, walking briskly. The water was smooth except when a little breeze made an occasional ripple. The trees looked dormant and wintry, although the afternoon was warm, and people filled the pedestrian and bike paths. Runners passed walkers. Cyclists barreled past or pedaled with comfortable ease, one pair of young women talking affably.

"Reminds me of us when we were college newbies," said Meg.

"Those days were fun," said Cate. "Few worries, few obligations."

On both sides of the pedestrian path, people rested on hammocks, reclined on blankets spread over brown grass, or picnicked; one couple grilled burgers on a hibachi, which emitted smells that reminded Cate of summer.

"Do you want to sit?" asked Meg.

"Not yet. Let's keep moving."

The two women slowed their pace and reminisced about their college days and twenty-year friendship. They'd met as freshmen violinists in the University of Pennsylvania orchestra, Meg an urbane doctor's kid from New Jersey, Cate an eager teen who'd never left St. Louis except for family trips to Florida in the summer, when rates were cheap. In their sophomore year, they shared a small apartment. They lived there through Penn graduate school as Cate cobbled together an interdisciplinary curriculum in psychology and business and Meg attended law school. Then Penn offered each of them faculty positions, Cate as an organizational psychologist at Wharton, the Penn business school, Meg teaching business ethics at the law school, and they moved to more sumptuous digs.

"God, who'd have thought both of us would end up in Minnesota," said Meg. "Two academics married to Minnesota guys, living the suburban life."

"That's on you," said Cate.

"Nope, it's on both of us. We always wanted to live in the same city."

Meg came first to the University of Minnesota, recruited by the law school. Shortly after that, she saw a posting to teach organizational psychology at the Carlson School of Management and called Cate, who applied and got the job. Once in Minneapolis, Cate, still an amateur violinist, auditioned for the Civic Orchestra of Minneapolis—

she loved the sensation of a violin beneath her chin, the magnificence of orchestral music—but Meg put her violin in the closet.

They walked quietly for a while, then race-walked a quarter of a mile, trudged another quarter mile in silence, found a bench, and sat watching the activity around them. Cate looked glum but said nothing.

"I thought we came here to talk about you and Jeff," said Meg.

"We did, but it's hard." Cate glared at the lake. "I hate being angry at him, but I'm constantly pissed. And I don't want to have the fight it would take to get past recriminations."

"That still astonishes me."

"Over the past year, I've grown a lot less tolerant when he doesn't listen. Instead of addressing it, I get angry and withdraw, but he doesn't address it either. We're faking it for the kids."

"You're the one that tells me to address conflict directly."

"I've gotten compliant. I adjust my weekend plans to accommodate him. He wants a ski vacation over winter break, and I say yes, so we're planning on Aspen instead of Sanibel."

"Then something's changed. You didn't start out that way."

"It takes too much effort. Shit, I have a colleague who listens better than Jeff."

"Who's that?"

"Jack Ross. You've heard me talk about him before."

"Your mentor? The conservative dude who hates affirmative action?"

"There's more to him than that. He's a good collaborator who respects my intellect. Besides, he's funny and interesting," said Cate.

"Uh-oh. That's what you used to say about Jeff."

"It's nothing like that. He lost his wife a year ago, and we started to talk more. Some afternoons we run together on the indoor track at the Fieldhouse."

"You talk about his wife?"

"A little about me. I try not to bring personal life to work."

"Back in college, we said we'd ask each other hard questions at important times," said Meg. "Remember?"

"Like two years ago, when you had that affair with a colleague?"

"Exactly, and I stopped because you asked hard questions. I realized I was being stupid and addressed the problems in my marriage. Think about it. You're getting something from that friendship that you should be getting from Jeff. You're not having an affair, but you might be on the way."

"Don't worry. I'd never do that." Cate looked at the lake, where a couple in down vests paddled a canoe, rounded an island, and disappeared. The wind stopped, and the lake seemed dark and flat. "Although I did tell him that Jeff and I have grown apart."

"Bad idea. Either you have that fight, or your marriage will fall into the chasm."

"You don't pull your punches, do you."

"Neither did you when I needed it. You're drifting, and you have to make a conscious choice, like the strong woman you are."

"I'm not feeling strong, but tell me, what choice would a strong woman make?"

"First, she'd think long and hard; she'd weigh her options. She might see a therapist or have a real heart-to-heart with her best friend, a whole lot more than you've told me so far. She would never leave because it seemed easier."

"Yeah. If she had the gumption, she'd have the goddamn fight." A gust rippled the water.

"Since when do you lack gumption?"

"I don't know. Maybe I should be angry at myself for pussyfooting around." Cate's eyes narrowed. "I'd never forgive myself if I ran away."

"There you go. That's the Cate I know."

"Let's walk some more," said Cate. "In fact, are you up for a sprint?"

"Sure."

They started with a gallop, then jogged at an easier pace part way around the lake, reversed direction, and jogged back toward the car. They found a bench and sat again, watching ducks that stayed the winter.

"When do you think you'll talk to him?" asked Meg.

"We planned to talk sometime after the holiday. It's funny, but I don't feel as desperate as I did before we talked. It's a good thing because I love Thanksgiving. It was always a fun time for me growing up."

"I like it too. It doesn't carry the weight of Christmas. Fewer family pressures."

"Usually," said Cate, returning Meg's grin. "Let's walk to the car and talk about tomorrow."

CHAPTER THREE:

Thanksgiving

Jeff carved the turkey as Cate, Meg, and Karen, Jeff's mom, set the rest of the food on platters atop the kitchen island, including the corn pudding that Jeff and his dad had put together that morning. Dan, with the four children and Jeff watching, had finished smoking the pecan pie. He looked with satisfaction at the pie and corn pudding, grinned at the children, and thumped Jeff on the shoulder.

At the dining room table, Kayla poured wine for the adults and Ben filled water glasses with the help of Evie and David. Then Kayla and Evie carefully lit four thick white candles, each surrounded by fall gourds. The centerpiece was a cornucopia filled with fruit and nuts and autumn-colored flowers accented with deep red and purple. Cate examined the table and smiled. Jeff, who did the dishes, wanted to use thick plastic plates from Costco, but Cate had insisted on her mother's bone china, Wedgwood, with a wide band of parchment and a gold rim.

First the children, then the adults, picked up their plates and, at the kitchen island, heaped food onto them and carried them to the table. Dan cautioned the children to be careful with the china, and Karen, with a head shake, winked at Cate. Jeff and Cate sat at the head and foot of the table. The rest sat wherever they landed, the children avoiding places with wine.

As everyone enjoyed their first bites of food, the table fell silent. Then pleasant chatter began. Scott asked Cate about her symposium. "Meg told me it's important."

"It's scheduled for late January and going very well."

"It's about leadership?"

"How transformational leaders respond to globalization. With an international faculty and, so far, over a hundred registrants." Cate's collaborator, Jennifer Land, had helped determine the structure and content of the conference, with suggestions from Jack Ross, their senior colleague.

"Jeff helped, too," said Cate. "He understands leadership and made excellent suggestions."

"Challenge and change. Cate loves to immerse herself in turmoil," said Jeff, with pride.

"Only at work," said Meg, with a knowing glance at Cate.

"That's right," said Jeff. "Cate's like Flaubert, regular and orderly in life, violent and original in work. I love that about her."

"Does that mean a regular and orderly marriage?" Scott laughed.

"I hope you know you married a tiger," said Meg. "Cate is about to make full professor."

"I do, and I couldn't be prouder."

After dessert, with empty plates stacked in the kitchen, some in soapy water, they retired to the family room. By the time Jeff's parents had departed with enough Thanksgiving leftovers to last a week, Cate still felt pleasantly stuffed. Ben and his friend David played in the basement, Kayla and Evie amused themselves in Kayla's room upstairs, and the four remaining adults relaxed in the family room where a fire crackled behind glass doors.

"That fire smells good," said Meg.

"It shouldn't smell." Jeff sniffed and walked to the fireplace. "I have to adjust those doors."

"We've all heard the lecture about fine particles and toxic gases in smoke," said Cate.

"It's even worse for children," said Jeff. "I'm taking care of our families."

"That much I appreciate," said Cate.

"Hey, who wants to watch Houston at Detroit?" said Scott, checking his watch. Neither the Vikings nor Packers had Thanksgiving games that year.

Cate and Meg left the football violence to the men and withdrew to the four-season porch, a peninsula surrounded on three sides by tall windows that made the landscape part of the room and served as an eating area and extra living space. Beyond the windows, boulders and evergreens rose above brown mulch, and oaks pushed into a gray and cloudy sky. Wicker furniture with bold black and white patterned cushions, accented with bright patterned pillows, and sun streaming through the windows made the porch airy and inviting.

"I've always loved this porch," said Meg.

"It's our favorite space," said Cate.

"If you want to preserve it, you have to bring that tiger home."

Cate looked toward the family room, where the TV blared. "When I think about what's good in the marriage and what's best for the kids, it's hard to make waves. I love the way he encourages my work and helps me think it through."

"He is good at that. But he does want you to be orderly at home. You do have happy kids, so I see the dilemma."

"When I was a kid, my parents screamed at each other a lot, especially after my sister died. I don't want that kind of home."

"And you kept the peace because screaming never solved anything. I'm talking about an argument with resolution, and you know very well how to do that. It fascinates me that you built a career managing conflict in others but avoid it at home."

"At work, it comes easy." Cate stared through the window at the yews—still green but dulled by fall. She steered the conversation to kids, school, shopping, and clothes, but the gears of her mind continued to grind.

Then she set her jaw and fixed her eyes on Meg. "Okay, I know you're right," said Cate. "I'll do it. I'll have that goddam fight."

CHAPTER FOUR:

Saturday

Two days after Thanksgiving, Cate and Jeff had not yet talked. In midafternoon, the door from the mudroom burst open as Cate and the children returned from the movies. The kids rushed onto the porch, where Jeff sat working on a project. "Robot & Frank was a good movie, Dad," said Ben. "Will you watch it with us sometime on TV?"

"Sure. What's it about?"

"Frank's son gave him a robot butler to look after him, but Frank trained it to help him steal things."

"Really?" Jeff looked at Cate, his face a question.

"It won the feature film prize at Sundance because it showed how dementia changed Frank's world," said Cate. "You'd enjoy it."

"Frank liked the librarian," said Kayla, "so he stole an old copy of *Don Quixote* from the library to get close to her."

"Sounds like something for everyone," said Jeff, laughing. "I'd love to watch it with you."

Cate motioned toward the back hall. The kids hung their coats on mudroom hooks and walked to the family room. Jeff left his project on the porch and joined them. Kayla picked up a book and sat next to Jeff on the couch; he put his arm around her, and she snuggled closer. Ben burrowed into his other side. Jeff gave them each an affectionate squeeze, picked up the *New York Times,* and they all read for a half hour while Cate prepared a snack and worked on dinner.

"Hey, does anyone want to play Roughhouse?" asked Jeff.

"Hooray," said Ben. He jumped up and ran to chairs with the beige snow leopard print near the family room windows. Kayla followed on his heels. Jeff perched on the love seat opposite the windows. Cate came from the kitchen to watch the game and took the couch on the side wall that faced the fireplace. Behind her hung a United Nations lithograph with four colorful busts of men and women, skin tones of black, yellow, red, and white, which floated in its frame like a harmonious Mount Rushmore. On the coffee table, a thin bronze figure carried a massive half circle of red-toned iron, *Burden of Deception*, a prize-winning student sculpture from the Minneapolis College of Art and Design. All these things, including the books and knickknacks on shelves on both sides of the fireplace, she and Jeff had collected over the years.

As Jeff leaned forward with arms outstretched, Ben yelled, "Yay, Roughhouse!" He ran across the room and launched his body into the air at Jeff, who caught him, used Ben's momentum to carry him to his chest for a hug, and placed Ben gently on his back. Kayla followed while Ben scurried away.

"Catch me, Dad," she cried.

After several launches, the kids needed a pit stop.

"Cate, do you want to try a launch?" asked Jeff, grinning, still on the couch.

"No thanks," said Cate. "You couldn't handle me."

"Bet I could."

"I'll leave it to the kids. They love this game, and they love you," said Cate.

"I love them too."

The kids returned and resumed the game. When their interest flagged, Jeff offered to read to them or play a board game and asked them to pick out something they both liked. Kayla and Ben raced up the stairs.

"They do love you, Jeff. Enjoy it while you can. Kayla's a tween who still likes spending time with you," said Cate.

"At least Ben's got a few more years."

"Speaking of Ben, have you noticed how he clings to you? He's always needed you in a special way. Even as a newborn, he wouldn't stop crying until you held him." Jeff nodded. "Besides that, he never seems satisfied with anything he does lately. And that nervous tic, tapping, always twice."

"He does seem anxious. I'll make it a point to spend more time with him."

"The movies would have been more fun with you there."

"Sorry I missed it. You know that December starts my busy season making cow embryos, and I have to prepare. Roughhouse was fun, and I have plans for both kids this weekend if we can work it out with your schedule. For one thing, they want to learn more about my work." Two weeks ago, Kayla and Ben visited Jeff's lab and, since then, have asked many questions about frozen embryos.

"I'll make it work."

"Don't forget how much time I spend with Ben and Quarter Midgets." Ben, his friend David, and both dads raced each weekend at Elko Speedway from late spring through October. Besides the races, there was maintenance and preparation. After each racing day, Ben helped his dad pull the racer from the trailer, remove the tires, and place the chassis on its stand inside the garage. The following week, before the races, they replaced the tires, tightened and adjusted the bearings, and retuned the engine. Ben learned to change or replace the valve springs, clean and adjust the carburetor, set the piston rings, reassemble the engine, and top off hydraulic fluid and fuel. Ben focused on the details, loving how the car went together, the smells of the engine, the sound when the engine ran smoothly, the smoothness of the chassis, and the comfort of sitting in the driver's seat and feeling the car respond to him as he drove.

Last month, once the racing season ended, Jeff helped Ben place the chassis on its stand. They worked together, deflating the tires, spraying them with Armor All to keep them pliable, carrying them to the basement for the winter, and resting them on their rims to avoid flat spots. Ben wiped surface dirt off the chassis.

Jeff planned to complete that winterizing later this afternoon and invited David and his dad to help. Last weekend, they'd winterized David's car.

"Embryos and racers. All good plans," said Cate.

* * *

Two years ago, when Ben and David were six, their dads suggested racing Quarter Midgets, cars that hurtled around a 1/20-mile track at thirty miles per hour, a sport for kids five to sixteen. Although racers wore safety equipment and cars had roll cages, waivers cited the risk of injury or death, but gymnastics, which the girls did, had the same waiver.

On a warm spring day in April two years ago, with trees beginning to leaf, the two families drove to Elko for the annual "Try it You'll Like It" event. Brightly colored cars filled the track and surrounding work areas as parents helped kids prepare for races. When a car spun out and sideswiped another, parents hurried onto the track to be sure the racers were not injured, and the involved cars drove into the race pit for a mandatory safety check. Cate put a stick of gum in her mouth and chewed vigorously.

Ben and David climbed into cars that belonged to other children, donned safety equipment, and took trial runs, one car at a time, around the track. Ben's glow of excitement hooked Cate and David showed the same enthusiasm. Kayla and Evie, although eligible to race, decided to stick with gymnastics and dance classes. By May, the dads had purchased used racers from the Quarter Midget website. Ben and David studied how the engines worked, the safety equipment, the flags the adults used to control the race, and racing rules. The sport emphasized safety and judgment.

Quickly, Ben learned to drive aggressively, how to swoop in from the outside, taking advantage of a slope on a curve, and drop to the inside, taking and holding the lead.

Early in their second year of racing, a car sideswiped Ben's car, which did a one-eighty and struck the car behind him head-on. Cate and Jeff ran to Ben, who said he was fine but searched for the race pit, confused. Cate insisted that they go to the ER, and the doctor admitted

Ben overnight for observation. This sent Cate to the internet; an article described a Florida accident where an ambulance crew had to use the Jaws of Life to extricate the driver, whose concussion symptoms lasted an entire week. Yet no parent who witnessed that accident kept his child from future races; "safer than football" was a common refrain. It took the boys and their dads two weeks to convince Cate and Meg to let them continue to race. For the rest of the racing season, Cate sat as close to the track as possible, and Meg sat beside her.

* * *

On the Saturday after Thanksgiving, the boys and dads removed the tarps from Ben's racer and carried it with its stand to the driveway. With the dads instructing, Ben and David drained the hydraulic fluid and fuel. Then they sprayed Simple Green degreaser on the engine and scrubbed it with a nonmetallic brush. "Use that elbow grease," said Jeff. The boys took turns. Then they wiped it dry with old rags.

"Are you satisfied?" asked Scott. The boys nodded.

"Time to hose it down," said David.

"First, we have to tape and cover the carburetor and exhaust to protect the openings," said Ben.

"You got it," said Jeff. The dads helped apply tape and plastic cloth. Then the boys hosed the engine, wiped it dry, finished the drying with an air compressor, and removed the protective materials.

"Okay, what's next?" asked Jeff.

"The chassis," said Ben. He used laundry detergent to scrub the magenta and bright blue fiberglass body, dried it gently with a cloth, and used the air compressor to dry it further. Then, carefully, he touched up the paint.

"It looks really nice," said David. The dads agreed.

"Thanks," said Ben. He examined the car and grinned.

After a break for snacks, allowing the paint to dry, they removed the engine from the chassis, wrapped it in plastic to prevent rodents from nesting inside during the winter, removed the shocks and batteries, checked the brakes, and coated the rear disks with WD-40 to avoid rust.

"Hey, Mom, come look," Ben shouted. Proudly, he described each step of what they had done.

"Nice job!" Cate said. "You boys earned another piece of pie."

The boys and dads washed up and gathered around the porch table.

CHAPTER FIVE:

Sunday

Seated on thick gymnastic mats that covered the floor of the finished basement, Kayla and her mom began with stretches. They gripped the fingers of one hand with the other, flexed and extended each wrist, holding each position, moved the wrist from side to side, and changed hands. Still seated, with one knee bent, then the other, they gripped their feet and pressed their ankles in every direction. On hands and knees, supine, on their sides, and finally standing, they stretched their backs, sides, and hips. Once limber, they did a few forward and backward rolls.

At 5' 8", Cate was tall for a gymnast but had competed through high school and continued tumbling for fun after she began long-distance running in college. She liked the discipline of gymnastics, its precision and control, and was glad that Kayla liked it too.

From a pile of CDs, Kayla selected *Where Them Girl At.* To the music, she did a handstand and walked a circle on her hands, followed by a forward roll, a few dance moves, and two forward flips, the last one a double. Cate applauded. "You make it look like fun."

"I'm lucky," Kayla teased. "The fun genes come from Dad."

"Thanks a lot." Cate managed a laugh and duplicated Kayla's run, omitting the double flip.

"Nice, Mom," said Kayla. "Now do it again with the double flip."

"Not sure I can."

"You're always telling me to push myself."

"Not beyond your capacity."

"You looked like you had some juice left. You don't know your limits until you try."

"Uh-oh. My own words are coming back to haunt me."

Kayla stood with her hands on her hips, grinning.

Cate retreated to the corner of the room, took a deep breath, then another, started with the handstand, and repeated the run. She managed two forward flips at the end, both singles.

"At least you tried, mom. Your second flip didn't look as clean."

"I could feel it. That's why I didn't try the double."

"Here's an easier one for you." Kayla did a cartwheel and a backward handspring and landed with a smile.

Cate imitated her but couldn't hold the landing and ended up on her butt, laughing. "Okay, honey, I admit it. You've gotten better than me."

"That's because I practice every day. Never miss. Just like you say."

"It might be that you're eleven, and I'm pushing forty."

"Mom, you're in great shape. It's just that you like marathons better than gymnastics. It wouldn't take too much practice to land that double flip if you really wanted it."

"I like your spirit, honey. Let's keep at it." They practiced together for over an hour. At the end of the time, Cate started in one corner and, with the help of forward motion, did a double flip. "How did that look?"

"Perfect."

"Guess I can do a double flip without a lot of stuff beforehand."

"Stuff? Please use better words."

"You're on me today. Is that what I really sound like?"

"Yup."

Cate frowned.

"But don't feel bad, Mom; it's fun to push myself. I like being good at what I do."

They climbed the stairs and collapsed on the couch in the family room as Ben and his dad finished a game of chess. Jeff flipped on the TV and found *Murder on the Orient Express* about to start. "Here's a good movie. Let's all watch it."

"Mom was gonna teach me how to make the meatballs for dinner," said Kayla.

"This is a busy family," said Jeff. "Too busy. Sometimes it's good to chill."

"Maybe Dad's right. We don't always have to be doing something productive, but Ben doesn't need to learn about murders."

"It's a mystery, Mom," said Ben. "I know about mysteries."

"I'll explain what he doesn't understand," said Kayla.

* * *

After supper and cleanup, Kayla and Ben looked eagerly at Jeff. "You promised to teach us more about your work," said Ben.

"You guys go. I have work to do," said Cate.

"Thanks," said Jeff with a smile.

Cate walked down the hall to her home office to get her computer.

Her desk drawer beckoned.

She hesitated because she was feeling good but opened the drawer and removed a yellow pad of paper. On the top sheet, she had scrawled separation/divorce, and below that had listed pros and cons.

Cate dropped heavily into the chair and considered them. The cons were easy. Failure of a twelve-year relationship, loss of a marriage that once felt magical. Moves, probably for both of them, with the loss of a house they loved, the only house the kids had known. Disruption for the kids, two households, complicated schedules and relationships. Harder to manage family/careers/school. Financial stress. Fleeing the marriage without confronting Jeff. Loss of a dream.

The pros felt more amorphous. Ending a marriage that didn't satisfy. Escape from anger and disappointment. Opportunity for a fresh start. Freedom to explore new relationships. She stared at the pros and tried to give them shape.

Her thoughts turned to Jack Ross. She enjoyed talking to him, liked working with him, felt respected, and adored the way he talked about his deceased wife. Sometimes, when she thought about him, she wondered if they could have a relationship. Was Jack catalyst or opportunity? Excuse or crutch?

Cate put the pad back in the desk drawer and closed it. She opened her computer but couldn't concentrate. She walked to the dining room door and observed Jeff and the kids. Kayla and Ben sat on either side of their dad.

"Imagine we're partners, and our job is to make the best milk," Jeff was saying. "What's in milk that makes it good?"

Ben guessed protein. Kayla, who had learned about milk at school, added butterfat and sugar and knew that milk was mostly water. Jeff patted their backs.

Cate smiled at the interaction. Jeff made everything feel like fun, and the kids worshipped him. She thought about the yellow pad and winced.

Jeff showed them a pie chart puzzle with three wedges: one for 87 percent water, another for 12 percent milk solids—protein, butterfat, and lactose—and a tiny 1 percent for vitamins and minerals. He removed all the wedges to focus on milk solids. Where the 12 percent wedge had been, Jeff substituted separate wedges for lactose, butterfat, and protein and asked what would make milk better. Ben guessed more protein. Kayla suggested butterfat.

Jeff applauded and showed them slightly larger wedges for protein and butterfat. He explained that the best milk had 20 percent more fat and 13 percent more protein, a big difference for growing kids. The pie chart made the differences easy to see.

"But how can milk from different cows be different?" asked Ben. "Cows all look the same."

"Take a close look at the picture of this herd and pay attention to the black and white spots," said Jeff.

"Hey, they're all different, like giraffes," said Ben.

"If spots can be different, milk can too," said Jeff.

Cate smiled. She felt drawn to Jeff as he worked with the kids.

She recoiled at the thought of hurting any of them.

"How do you get cows to give the best milk, Dad?" asked Ben.

"Remember those embryos we saw in my lab?" said Jeff.

"We looked at them with a microscope," said Kayla.

Jeff showed them, with diagrams and pictures, how he injected sperm through a plastic tube into the uterus of a cow. After a week, he washed the embryo out of the cow's uterus into a petri dish, froze the embryo with liquid nitrogen, and placed it in the freezer.

"How do you know which cows to use?" asked Ben.

"We find a cow who gives good milk. Then we breed the father of that cow with other cows who give good milk. We breed them until the milk gets better and better."

Kayla worried that freezing and unfreezing might hurt the embryos. Ben remembered dad's banana trick. In his lab, they had dipped a banana into liquid nitrogen, used the frozen banana to pound a nail, thawed the banana, and ate it. "That banana tasted good." Ben rubbed his tummy.

Cate laughed. "If you're hungry, I have cake and some of Dad's best milk." They adjourned to the kitchen and snacked.

Back at the table, Jeff said, "Okay, now that I have these embryos, what do I do with them?"

"You send them to farms where kids need better milk," said Ben.

"Dad has to put the embryos back inside cows to grow into calves," said Kayla.

"You're both right. Wherever we send the embryos, someone has to insert them into a cow's uterus."

"Because cows are just like us," said Kayla.

"Yeah," said Ben. "They have to grow inside a mother."

Cate could not resist a smile. When the kids first asked how babies were made, Cate had pulled out her ragged copy of *A Baby is Born, The Story of How Life Begins,* a Golden Book from the 1940s passed down from Cate's grandmother to her mother to Cate. The book, well ahead of its time, said that a father and mother lie close together, the penis enters the vagina, and, with diagrams of tadpole-like sperm growing in testicles and swimming in semen, eggs growing in ovaries, described fertilization, growth, and birth.

"I want to help you make embryos when I'm older," said Ben.

"Mom says your lab's a business that helps farmers," said Kayla. "I don't like cows, but I could help with the business part."

"You're right. My lab is a business. Did you know that farming is a business, too?"

"I guess farmers want the best milk because they can sell it for more money," said Kayla.

"That's right. There's a lot that happens before that gallon of milk gets to the grocery store."

Cate thought about all that Jeff had not described—computer chips with genetic information embedded in the neck of every cow, automated pails that analyzed milk and sent butterfat and protein data to the chip, the use of bulls and cows from different herds to avoid inbreeding, bulls worth $250,000 that fertilize 60,000 cows in a lifetime, the use of "donor cows" good at bearing calves and prepped with hormones. And there was the newer process of in vitro fertilization—washing eggs instead of embryos from the uterus, fertilizing eggs in a petri dish, and growing the embryos for a week in that dish before freezing.

Cate sighed. She loved that Jeff was on the cutting edge. She had always loved that about him. She cherished the way Jeff engaged the children, the way they hung on his words. Loving the kids and sharing that love enriched her relationship with Jeff. But was that enough to sustain a marriage?

* * *

After the kids were in bed, Cate sat on the loveseat next to Jeff, feeling a bit closer to him after watching him with the kids. All the décor—from the snow leopard chairs to the gray leather couch and love seat, to the Sherwin-Williams mellow yellow walls, to every painting and all the objects found at art fairs or on trips, the large raku vase, the globe from China inset with variegated stones—they had chosen together.

"I love this room," said Cate.

"Me too," said Jeff. "It's been fun adding things over the years."

"We did that well," she said. "We still do some things pretty well. Responsibility for the kids. Schedules. Anything with structure."

"I know," said Jeff, his face sad. "We've lost the fun of it. I'd like to get that back."

"I would, too," said Cate. "At least I think so."

"You *think* so?"

"The only reason schedules work is that I make all the accommodations," said Cate.

"That's not true. We treat each other as equals."

"Sometimes it feels like equal foxholes, and I give in. You want everything your way, even vacations."

"That's because you never want to go anywhere fun."

"It's not just vacations," said Cate.

Jeff cocked his head.

"You're listening now, but too often it feels like you're not." Cate kept her voice calm, but her lips thinned, and her nostrils flared.

"You look like you're pissed, but you don't sound like it."

"I want to have a conversation, not an argument."

"For God's sake, if you're angry, show it. That fake calm is chilling." Jeff's face reddened, and his voice grew harsh.

"Don't talk like that to me."

"At least it's authentic. I want to hear what else is bugging you. Then I'll give you my list."

"*Your* list?"

"Let's clear the air. You used to love a good fight. We've stopped fighting about important things."

"The children might be awake. I don't want them to hear."

"You don't want to engage. Look, I admit that I haven't either. We can have an honest fight without yelling and screaming, but you can't hide inside your shell. *That's* not good for the kids, who sure as hell know we're not getting along. It's making them like you, afraid of conflict."

"What bullshit. I study conflict for a living."

"At home, you're afraid of your own shadow."

Cate gulped. Meg had made a similar observation. "Will you

please talk softly? I told you I don't want to scare the kids."

"Come on, Cate. They know. They're already scared."

"Kayla isn't scared," said Cate. "She says what's on her mind."

"We're both worried about Ben."

"He's anxious, but not because of us."

"You don't know that," said Jeff. "And you can't count on things staying calm with Kayla. You can't handle a rebellious teenager."

Cate glared at Jeff and stomped out of the family room.

"That's what I'm talking about," Jeff called after her. "You run away."

"That's a stupid comment," said Cate, on the way to the kitchen.

When she returned with a cup of hot tea, Jeff added a birch log to the fire, watched it catch, and added a second one. "When did you become such a milquetoast?" he said. "On our Cape Town honeymoon, you insisted we hike to the top of Table Mountain. You said it would be more fun than the cable car. You wanted the challenge."

"The Cape of Good Hope, Stellenbosch wine country, Robben Island. I did love that trip," said Cate.

"So did I."

"Look, I know I haven't been the same lately. For one thing, I haven't been sleeping well. I'm worried about us."

"Are you having those nightmares again, like the ones you had after Kayla was born?"

Cate's eyes widened. "How did you know?"

"You're acting the way you did then—irritable and critical of me. It feels the same."

"Those nightmares scare me."

"They didn't stop until you figured out they were related to Sally's death."

Cate stared at the burning logs. "They came back this past winter. I used to dream that something happened to Kayla. Now it's both of them."

"Eleven," said Jeff.

"What?"

"Sally was eleven when she died. Kayla will turn eleven in February. Maybe that's what's bothering you."

When Cate was twelve, and her sister was eleven, Sally wore one of Cate's dresses to school without permission. On the bus ride home, Cate screamed at her. When they got off the bus, Cate chased her, and Sally ran into the street in front of a passing car. Cate watched her sister catapult through the air. She cradled her, bleeding from the head, until she disappeared into the ambulance, and two days later, Sally died. Cate had nightmares for more than a year. Shortly after Kayla's birth, the nightmares returned.

Cate paced for several minutes before she sank again into the couch beside Jeff. "That might contribute to what's going on because I feel a little better thinking about it, putting it together. Sometimes you amaze me."

"Would it help to talk more?" Cate had rarely talked to Jeff about Sally's death and the aftermath, except to say it was the worst time of her life. Her parents fought or sat in stony silence.

"Mom shut me down because every time I mentioned Sally, my dad erupted. I had thoughts of running into a car and dying like Sally. If it hadn't been for the school counselor, who knows?"

"That's horrible."

"The part you don't see is that *you* shut me down when you don't listen."

"I'll think about that. I really will." He took a deep breath and blew it out. "But I can't be responsible for your reactions."

"Fuck you, Jeff."

"Okay. That was a dumb comment, and I'm sorry." He reached for her. She did not pull away, unsure how all the threads of her life fit together.

At half past ten, they climbed the stairs together, looked in on the sleeping kids, and Jeff put an arm around Cate. They brushed their teeth at matching sinks and, for the first time in a week, did not crawl to opposite edges of their king-size bed.

CHAPTER SIX:

Monday after Thanksgiving

In the mudroom, Cate removed her fleece jacket and unlaced her black running shoes as the grandfather clock, a wedding present from her parents, pealed the sixteen notes of the Westminster chimes followed by seven resonant gongs. She tramped into the kitchen, still breathing hard, makeup-free, and flushed by the cold November air. Her dark blue running suit, splashed with red, followed the contours of her figure, which last night, she thought with a smile, had moved with lithe energy beneath Jeff. She headed for the porch. At the table, four bowls of oatmeal rested on placemat souvenirs from their Cape Town honeymoon, with sparsely sketched elephants dancing on banners of burgundy, rust, and blazing orange. Cate smiled at Jeff and the kids.

"How was your run?" asked Jeff.

"Getting there. I'm almost ready." In a couple of weeks, they planned a weekend trip to Dallas, where Cate would run the Dallas Marathon. She tried to run two marathons a year, one in Minnesota and one somewhere else. It was easy to get away as a couple, with Jeff's parents only an hour away and glad to look after the kids, but this time they planned to take Kayla and Ben.

"We're gonna cheer for you at the finish line," said Kayla.

"I'll wave if I still have energy."

"Maybe we should watch Mom at the start of the race," said Jeff.

"No! The end!" said Ben.

"Okay." Cate laughed. "I promise to wave." She glanced at the kitchen clock. It was late. She hurried the kids into their coats. Quick kisses, and they were gone.

Usually, Jeff dashed off to make embryos well before the kids left. Instead, he filled two cups with coffee, pushed the skim milk toward Cate, and asked about the symposium. Cate replied that it was coming along, except for a thousand loose ends. Jeff offered to get the kids off to school every morning that week to ease the load of preparing for the symposium and training for the race instead of taking turns getting the kids out the door.

"Thanks, honey." She hesitated. "Jeff, I appreciate what you're doing, but we still need to talk."

"About the symposium?" He grinned.

"About everything. Your observation about Sally helped, but I'm still angry."

"Then let's keep talking, but you have to acknowledge that we both contribute."

"Dammit, Jeff, if you just accepted my invitation and listened, we'd get to your concerns."

"Right."

"Look, can't you see I'm not withdrawing? I'm not hiding in my shell. What do you want?"

"You know what I want. I want you," said Jeff.

"No, you don't. You feel good about yourself when you admire my work and when you do your part at home, but you want a compliant wife who doesn't rock the boat."

"Bullshit. I don't want you to be compliant."

"You *do*. It looks like equality, but it's not, dammit." Cate stomped upstairs to the shower.

Jeff followed her to the bedroom and waited until she had dried herself and dressed.

"I want to keep talking," he said

"It's time for work. I'm busier than hell."

"Is the symposium part of what's getting to you?"

"First Sally. Now the symposium. Everything contributes, but they're not the problem."

"Then what is?"

"You."

"I'll think about that."

"Good, and I'll think about what you said."

CHAPTER SEVEN:

Sunday Evening, Six Days Later, and the following Morning

With the kids asleep, Jeff approached Cate as she prepared to put on her nightgown and stroked her arm. "You look lovely," he said. She knew Jeff liked the way subdued light from a single bedroom lamp made her skin dusky white, her breasts alluring, her firm abs and supple legs attractive. His touch aroused her, but the heat that burned with fury in her head surprised her. She turned so that her side faced him. The back meant something else. "Not now," she said, her voice husky.

Jeff, shirtless, wearing only underpants, reached for her and massaged her neck and shoulders. He scraped his fingernails gently against her neck, and her skin tingled. Cate, suspended between arousal and refusal, said again, "Not now," but she leaned into him. He pulled her close. With one hand still on her shoulder, he raised his other hand and his fingers played against her breasts, caressing her nipples in the way she liked. Her nipples grew hard, and she closed her eyes and enjoyed the warmth that spread upward to her face and down to her inner thighs. She swayed slightly at the hips and turned to face Jeff with her lips parted. He wrapped his arms around her waist and pressed his body against hers, increasing her excitement, although her fisted hands hung at her side. She raised her hands to his shoulders and pushed him away without stepping back, so their legs still touched, her ambivalence increasing both his arousal and hers.

"What's going on?" His voice was hoarse.

His need excited her; it made her eager for his touch, her mouth yearning to crush his lips, but she moved away and glared.

"I've never seen you like this. Are you turned on or pissed off?" asked Jeff.

"Both."

"If you're pissed, you have a nice way of showing it." She stood within reach and didn't move. Jeff wrapped both hands around the back of her head and kissed her; she pushed her tongue into his mouth and tasted him. He kissed her neck and shoulders, and she did the same, scraping him with her teeth, pushing his head against her breasts, lifting her head in ecstasy. But she stepped back, breathing quickly, hands gripping his shoulders, holding on but keeping him at arm's length.

Jeff stared at her.

"Maybe I don't want to do this," she said, and shoved him, taking charge. She took a step forward and shoved him again. "Does this piss you off? I hope so because I'm boiling." They each held their ground, inches from each other, until Cate closed the distance between them, kissed his neck, moved her lips and tongue against his ear and then his mouth, enjoying the feel of his hardness against her, his urgency, wanting and not wanting more. She dug her nails into his back and pulled him toward her, and they kissed hard. "You think I don't like risk, that I want everything safe and secure."

"You do."

His taunt enraged her. "Fuck you." She raised her palms to his chest and pushed him backward onto the bed, yanked off his underpants, and flicked her tongue against his thighs. She lifted his legs onto the bed, then climbed onto him, taking his fullness inside her, and moved until he moaned. Then she stopped moving and glared into his eyes. He thrust upward, but she resisted.

"Dammit, move," he said.

"When I'm ready."

She began to undulate, maximizing her own pleasure, teasing him, keeping him on the edge, using his excitement to fuel hers, feeling her ecstasy build until her clitoris exploded and wave after wave of fire coursed through her. Only then did she relieve him, making his spasms augment hers. She sank onto the bed beside him, and they lay there staring at each other, not touching. Jeff reached for her, but Cate shifted away.

"What the hell just happened?"

"You're lucky I'm not a praying mantis. I'd have bitten off your head."

"I'll give you that."

The release had freed something inside her. "Dammit, Jeff, I've been thinking about separation, really thinking."

"Somehow, that doesn't surprise me. Now that you said it, maybe we can both talk and both listen."

"Can't you stop telling me what to do?"

"We have to talk."

"What the hell do you think just happened? Wasn't that communication?"

"I liked it. I liked you. But it wasn't talking. Something keeps us from resolving things."

"It's *you,* goddamn it. *You* don't listen. *You* shut me down."

Jeff swallowed and said nothing.

"Good," said Cate. "Don't say a word." She yawned, suddenly exhausted, and turned her back to him. After several minutes, she rolled to face him. "Just shut up, and I'll see how I feel in the morning." She closed her eyes and eventually fell asleep.

* * *

Cate awoke Monday morning before the alarm on sheets crumpled from restless slumber, her back to Jeff. Outside, thick snow dripped through the first trace of morning light. She turned on her bedside lamp, rolled to look at Jeff, and found his eyes open. "How are you this morning?" he asked.

She touched his arm. "A lot less angry. It's been building for a while."

"We both let that happen. I'm sorry."

"Some of it's me," said Cate. She got out of bed and put on her short silk bathrobe, an October birthday gift from Jeff.

"I appreciate your saying that," said Jeff. He stood and stretched. "Do you have time this morning after the kids leave for school?"

"I want to talk, but I have a morning class to teach. Tonight, when we're not rushed?"

"Fitting 'us' into our schedules is part of the problem," said Jeff.

"I agree. But this talk can't be squeezed for time."

"It's a date," said Jeff, as he headed for the shower.

"A date. I remember those. Hurry up, and we can have breakfast before school," said Cate.

"Be right down," said Jeff.

Through the glass shower door, Cate watched him rub his body with soap. She tightened her robe and headed toward the children's rooms to be sure they were awake.

* * *

Downstairs, beyond the windows of the four-season porch, Cate watched the first storm of the season blossom into a windless blur, late this year on the first Monday in December. Heavy snow, made beautiful by the red-orange hues of early dawn, outlined the branches of hardwoods, pushed evergreens toward the ground, and carpeted the landscape. As predicted, the temperature had dropped precipitously, but the snowfall was supposed to stop in an hour or two. Cate dialed the Hopkins school line. No late start and no cancellation. Cate smiled. After all, this was Minnesota.

Ben arrived, eager to make a snowman after dinner. Kayla said she was too old for snowmen, but Jeff said she could use her gymnastic muscles to help roll the snow into balls. Cate had an old hat, buttons, carrots, and fruit. "You can both help make the face," she said.

Jeff glanced at his watch, brushed Cate's lips with his, kissed both kids on the forehead, rummaged through the mudroom closet for his parka, and hurried into the garage. From the family room windows, with a rush of tenderness, Cate watched Jeff's SUV descend the driveway.

The SUV faltered as it entered the roadway, slipped again as it negotiated a curve, and faded into the storm. Several minutes later, the school bus, a few minutes late, its headlights partially obscured by falling snow, appeared, then disappeared around the corner, negotiating the curve without slipping, the children safely inside.

Cate headed for the shower, her daily respite—her precious few minutes of solitude each day, when the children were on the bus and Jeff was on his way to work, before she left for the University. She tried to relax into the massage as warm pulses of water loosened taut muscles, aware that much remained unsettled.

CHAPTER EIGHT:

Jeff, the Same Morning, December 3

Jeff felt the car slide sideways as it left the driveway. He knew the snow had melted and frozen again, and the roads would be treacherous.

Past the slippery curve, he pulled over. For a moment, the day could wait. The snow, thick and falling, blanketed every surface with pristine loveliness. He opened a window and extended a gloved hand to catch a few crystals, savoring the frigid breeze that streamed across his face. Forty years old, and he still loved the dry smell of winter and the charm of a snowflake. He removed a glove and wiped a tear from his eyes, thinking of last night, the morning, and the future of his marriage.

What would I do without Cate? Without my family? he thought.

Twelve years ago, almost to the day, Jeff had walked through the carved oak doors of the Conrad Room at the downtown Minneapolis Hilton to attend a seminar about transformational leadership and encountered Cate at the head of the table—striking, slender, and fit, with dark brown hair, an oval face, and brown eyes penetrating and bright. He remembered how he tried not to blush. She looked about the same age as Jeff, in her late twenties, dressed in a camel blazer, white blouse and black slacks. As the seminar progressed, he liked the way she commanded the room and put others at ease.

"What are the qualities of a transformational leader?" she'd asked, with a smile that was confident and welcoming. She invited discussion and drew from the attendees the descriptions she wanted—vision, courage, tenacity, the capacity to inspire—and explored with authority the meaning of each quality. He found everything about her compelling.

Jeff approached her with a question, and she commented on the biography he had prepared for her seminar. His father had learned Quechua before going to Cuzco for the Peace Corps. Jeff had studied Fulfulde, the regional language of Burkina Faso, not the colonial French, before his own Peace Corps time. Jeff sensed mutual attraction. At least, he hoped he did. Discussion continued until they were alone. He invited her for coffee, and she accepted.

One week later, they met at the Purple Onion coffee shop near the university campus. Cate had liked his choice, one of the first places in the nation to voluntarily create a nonsmoking section. To Jeff's surprise, Cate had never visited Dinkytown, a four-block area adjacent to the campus. He enjoyed showing her this campus hotspot, crammed with bars, restaurants, bookstores, and mom-and-pop stores; the Purple Onion sat in its heart. Over the ensuing twelve years, Dinkytown, with its charm and personality, would become their special space, full of memories.

Jeff took in a breath of crisp, cold air and rolled up the window. With a last look at the billowy whiteness, he shifted into drive and pressed the accelerator. As he turned from his street onto the main road, two Hopkins police cars flashed red and blue lights alongside dented fenders. He skidded again. Three miles later, he entered the ramp onto northbound Highway 100, several car lengths behind a phalanx of snowplows barreling down the highway at forty miles per hour, a Minnesota trio spewing sand and salt, the leftmost plow in the lead, the other two successively behind to clear the road in a single pass. A pair of oncoming headlights separated from the southbound row of lights, found a gap between temporary barriers erected for road construction, entered his lane behind the snowplows, and aimed for him. In a panic, he crushed his foot against the brakes. Despite fresh sand and salt, his tires barely gripped the pavement. Trucks and cars filled every northbound lane. There was no escape. Jeff heard himself scream, then he registered the sound of crumpling metal before the head-on collision.

CHAPTER NINE:

Cate, the Same Morning

As Jeff drove to work, Cate allowed herself a longer-than-usual shower to think about the last twelve hours. By owning her anger and expressing it, she'd made room for tenderness, revived it. Feeling hopeful, she dried herself and used the towel to knead her neck and shoulders, arms and legs, building on the work done by the shower massage, enjoying the gentle burn of terrycloth on her skin. Outside the window, snowflakes illuminated by dawn light glistened with crystalline beauty.

She decided on a charcoal skirt, matching wool sweater, and an ivory blouse because, after teaching class, she had a meeting with the dean and department chair to discuss academic promotion. She anticipated no problems, especially since the dean had asked Cate to blurb her new book on corporate social responsibility and relate it to Cate's work on leadership. Satisfied that she looked professional but not too formal, Cate climbed into her Accord and drove cautiously through the diminishing snowfall to the university.

In the Nineteenth Avenue ramp, she began the hike toward her office. Always efficient, Cate extracted her iPhone from her gray leather shoulder bag and scanned it. There were two messages from Words with Friends, her games with friends Meg and Indra, who ran a consumer electronics retailer, and a slew of work-related emails and messages. It would be a busy morning. As she opened the door to the ramp stairs, the phone vibrated in her hand. She debated whether to answer or ignore it. The caller ID said HCMC, the hospital name on Hennepin County ambulances. She pressed the green icon, held it to her ear, and said hello.

"This is Betty Rogers, the charge nurse in the Emergency Department at HCMC. Your husband, Jeff Richards, is here." The words felt like a distant scream. "Are you driving?"

"No. I just parked in the ramp." With one hand on the door open to the stairs, she looked back at her car.

"Jeff had a car accident. Can you come to the hospital?"

"Yes, of course. I'm at the U, fifteen minutes away." She let the ramp door close and leaned against it. "How badly is he hurt?" A quiver began in her voice and surged through her body.

"The doctors are still evaluating him. We'll have a better idea by the time you get here."

"I'd like to know more about the accident. Is there anything else you can tell me?"

"We know he was unconscious at the scene and confused and restless when he got here. He has several fractures."

"What kind of fractures?"

"His face, ribs, maybe his pelvis, and probably his skull. The doctors have ordered CT scans and X-rays."

"God. He must be in pain."

"He's asleep and pain free. The doctors sedated him in part because he was too agitated to examine. Cate, it helps to have support. Can you ask a friend or family member to meet you here?"

"I'll call my friend, Meg."

Without noticing her steps, she hurried back to her car, opened the door, and leaned against it. She steadied her fingers, dialed Meg's cell, reached voice mail, and asked Meg to meet her at HCMC. She got in, started the car, backed out of her space, almost hit a passing car, and sped toward the ramp exit. At the first traffic light at Riverside and Cedar Avenues, on streets she knew well, Cate was not sure which route to take. She punched HCMC into Google Maps. At the next light on 3rd Street, she remembered her class and meeting and called the department office. The secretary wished her well and assured her she would get the class covered and cancel the meeting.

As her iPhone squawked directions, Cate fumbled with the radio and searched for traffic reports, hoping to learn something about what had happened. WCCO described an accident that had to be Jeff's. A car had crossed the median on Highway 100 in Golden Valley, collided head-on with an SUV, and flipped on its side, blocking all lanes of northbound traffic. The driver of the car died at the scene. An ambulance had taken the driver of the SUV, condition unknown, to HCMC. Cate gripped the steering wheel, trying to control her worry.

At the hospital, Cate parked where Betty had suggested, in the small lot outside the ER, spoke briefly to the security guard, raced through the double glass doors, and found another guard who directed her to the triage nurse who sat at a desk inside a large open window talking on the phone. For a few seconds, Cate shifted from foot to foot until the nurse cradled the phone.

"I'm Cate Richards. My husband …"

"I'm Jean. We're expecting you."

Cate nodded. The triage nurse hurried Cate on a tortuous path through emergency room corridors toward Betty and the stabilization room, where Jean said the ambulance delivered patients with trauma; Jean pointed to a row of chairs across the hall from wide double doors, pressed a button, and the automatic doors swung open. At the far end of a large space, Cate saw people move in what looked like a ghostly diorama. The doors closed behind Jean.

Cate waited, vaguely aware of a fetid smell of vomit emanating from the nursing station behind her. Her phone chimed, and a text said Meg was on the way.

Shortly, Jean emerged with Betty, a tall blonde nurse in green scrubs who managed a friendly smile, shook Cate's hand with a firm grip, and explained that the doctors would talk to her as soon as they completed their initial evaluation; Cate could see him in the stabilization room or wait. She asked if a friend or family member was coming and said a chaplain was available as well.

"A chaplain?" Cate's voice dropped to a whisper. "Is Jeff dying?"

"No," Betty answered quickly, "it's about support."

Cate wanted to see Jeff at once, without a chaplain, without waiting for Meg. Betty put a hand on Cate's shoulder and kept it there as she prepared Cate for what she'd see. Jeff was in an induced coma, free of pain, and unaware of the busyness around him.

As they walked through the doors and crossed the large space, a confusion of green and blue scrubs, bright lights, and machines with multicolored dials came gradually into focus. The scene felt otherworldly, macabre. At the center of the mayhem, a replica of Jeff lay on its back, its face bruised, covered by a blanket from the neck down, illuminated by a glaring surgical spotlight, enmeshed in tubes and wires that reminded Cate of a nest of snakes. One snake, connected to a respirator, filled his mouth and distorted his lips. Other devices, chirping and blinking, monitored blood pressure and vital signs. The dozen or so people that crowded around him were emergency room physicians, residents, nurses, technicians, medical students, note takers, and others. The tall, dark-haired man by Jeff's head was the emergency medicine physician in charge. The man examining Jeff's eyes was the neurosurgical resident.

"Did you say neurosurgeon?"

"Yes. With loss of consciousness, confusion, and a probable skull fracture, it's possible that Jeff has a traumatic brain injury."

Cate felt like she was drifting on a cloud. Her palms and face grew damp. The stabilization room was huge, much of it dark and empty and full of unused beds, which added to Cate's sense of unreality. *That can't be Jeff on the table,* she thought. *It's some kind of bizarre illusion.* She thought about the pleasant anticipation around the breakfast table and jammed her eyes shut. *Jeff is going to build a snowman with Ben and Kayla tonight in the front yard.*

"It's a lot to handle," said Betty. They were about to take Jeff for a CT scan of his brain and head, so Betty walked Cate back to the hallway to await the doctors. "There will likely be some decisions to make," said Betty.

The word exploded. "Decisions?"

"About Jeff's care. He might need surgery."

For an instant, Cate felt dizzy. Then her mind sharpened as she entered what she'd come to call her crisis mode, weighing and considering information safely in her head, making decisions as she did every day as an academic, channeling the febrile energy of panic into reason.

* * *

Meg leaped from her chair in the hallway to greet Cate, studied her at arm's length, and drew her in for a hug. Cate clung to Meg until her composure returned and she could bring Meg up to date: the accident, the stabilization room pandemonium, the induced coma, and what she knew so far about Jeff's injuries. It helped to talk.

Then the wide doors sprang open, and Betty and three doctors emerged. Cate introduced Dr. O'Reilly, the emergency room physician, who in turn introduced the staff neurosurgeon and his resident and hurried them toward a conference room a few steps down the hall. Cate and Meg matched their brisk pace.

As they entered the conference room, a great oak framed by a window on the far wall drew Cate's attention, its thick branches lined with mantles of white, stark against a background of red brick on the other side of a courtyard. The snow had stopped and the tree, glowing in the morning sun, thrust upward like Rodin's Monument to Balzac. Its solitary power seemed to fortify Cate.

"I'm sorry, but we have to talk quickly," said Dr. O'Reilly, who gestured toward two chairs. "Jeff's main problem is a traumatic brain injury. There's an urgent issue, so I want Dr. Watkins, the neurosurgeon, to go first."

Dr. Watkins spoke rapidly. His laptop displayed a CT image of Jeff's brain. He pointed to a crescent of dense white inside Jeff's skull, above his left ear, a large blood clot called a subdural hematoma, which would likely continue to bleed. Because the skull is like a rigid box with no room for escaping blood, bleeding can raise pressure inside the brain to dangerous levels, Dr. Watkins explained. He planned to drill a hole in Jeff's skull, suck out the clot, stop the vein from bleeding, and stick a monitor beneath the skull to be sure brain pressure stayed low.

On another CT image, he showed them dark areas deep within the brain, ventricles that hold spinal fluid, their shape distorted by pressure from the clot. A thin membrane in the center of the brain was shifted about 1 millimeter to the right, also indicating significant pressure. Dr. Watkins would insert a tube into the ventricles so they could remove spinal fluid to lower pressure if pressure increased suddenly from swelling or more bleeding in the next few days. The tiny tube would pass through brain tissue but not cause significant damage.

"What happens if you don't do all that?" asked Cate.

"The risks are brain damage and death from respiratory arrest," said Dr. Watkins.

Meg leaned forward. "When would you start?"

"As soon as Cate signs this consent form. He's already on his way to the operating room."

"What are the risks?" asked Meg, looking at the form.

"Infection and other kinds of bleeding, but the biggest risk is waiting."

Cate grabbed the form and scrawled a signature. Dr. Watkins and his resident rushed out the door with a promise to find Cate when they were done.

After they left, Dr. O'Reilly offered a warm, reassuring smile. "Subdurals are common, so they do this operation a lot." He paused. "Both of you look exhausted. How about a stretch to clear your heads? I can sure use one."

Cate stood and stretched her arms and legs. She walked to the window and stared at the Balzac tree before she returned to sit beside Meg, facing Dr. O'Reilly, eager for more information.

He began by opening his laptop to the same CT images. There was more to know about Jeff's traumatic brain injury, what he called a TBI, a term they would hear a lot. Cate fidgeted with the buttons on her sweater as she looked at images of her husband's brain. It was easy to see the skull fracture, a dark line that interrupted the smooth flow of bone on the left side of Jeff's forehead. Inside his skull, white spots indicated trouble. There was a brain contusion or bruise just below the skull fracture, on the left side of the brain, in what Dr. O'Reilly called the language area. There were many tiny hemorrhages scattered throughout Jeff's brain and a tiny right-sided subdural hematoma that would resolve on its own without surgery. Like bruises and hemorrhages anywhere in the body, Dr. O'Reilly explained, swelling would develop around them in the next few hours and days, increasing the pressure inside the rigid skull box, another reason for the pressure monitor.

Meg gripped Cate's hand.

"There's more we can talk about, other injuries besides the brain," said Dr. O'Reilly, "but not everyone wants this much information."

Cate wanted to know as much as possible. Dr. O'Reilly suggested another stretch.

She stood and again gathered strength from the Balzac tree. In addition to Meg, it seemed like her best friend. Betty fetched Styrofoam cups and a pitcher of ice water from the nearby nursing station. Cate pressed the ice against her teeth as Dr. O'Reilly continued.

He explained that Jeff had fractures of both cheekbones and bleeding into his left hip and buttock, but fortunately, no hip or pelvic fracture. A fractured rib on the left had collapsed a lung. To expand it, they had inserted a tube into his chest and connected it to a suction machine. That and the respirator helped him breathe.

Dr. O'Reilly raised his eyebrows, Cate nodded, and he pressed on.

The orbit, the bony sphere that held the eye, was fractured on the left side. Ophthalmology had examined him in the stabilization room; fortunately, the eye itself was intact, so it would also heal on its own; they would check it again in the operating room.

"That's it. Any questions?"

"How long before he's out of danger?" asked Cate.

"Once the subdural is gone, after surgery, he should do well, but they'll watch him very closely. In the first week or so, they'll likely remove the equipment that monitors and supports him. None of the injuries outside the brain would cause long-term problems."

"Then how long before he's back to normal?"

Dr. O'Reilly responded that HCMC had an excellent brain injury team that would help Jeff and her along the way. Cate pressed him, and Dr. O'Reilly said the details were beyond his expertise, but from experience, he thought weeks or months or longer. The contusion in the language area might mean he'd have trouble making or understanding speech, like some people with a stroke, and that usually improves in a few months. The main problem was the diffuse injury throughout the brain, and that might take longer to heal. "What I do know is that every brain injury is different, and you can't predict recovery from what you see in these pictures."

Cate swallowed hard.

"This is a huge amount of information to consider, way more than I usually provide at this juncture, but I let your questions guide me. First, let's get him safely through surgery."

Dr. O'Reilly stood, offered an encouraging smile, and suggested a cup of coffee or something cold to drink until they could see Jeff in the ICU. Betty told them where to find the ICU lounge and how to find the coffee shop and cafeteria.

CHAPTER TEN:

Cafeteria

Cate felt like she was watching herself in a silent movie—detached, looking down at herself from the cafeteria ceiling. She saw Meg lean close to her and speak, squeeze her arm until it blanched, but Cate heard or felt nothing. She watched, half awake, half dreaming, her head filled with poorly formed images—crescents of white beneath Jeff's skull, operating room surgeons gathered around his head, drilling bone.

Meg squeezed Cate's arm and rubbed, she squeezed and rubbed harder, she spoke loudly in Cate's ear. Gradually, Meg's familiar voice and persistent touch pulled Cate back into her body, to memories of last evening's anger-fueled passion, the morning hope of reconciliation, the image of Jeff as a replica sprouting tubes.

Cate saw people, blurred and indistinct, standing in cafeteria lines, moving about, or seated at tables. The people had faces, they had clothes with colors, bright or pastel, solid or patterned. She recognized the cafeteria smells of late morning, fried food and pizza colliding with eggs and waffles and coffee.

Meg looked at her. "How are you doing?"

"I don't know." Cate moved her arms and legs, she stood, she stretched her arms above her head, she sat and tried to clear her head.

"Tell me what you're worried about."

"Besides Jeff?"

"About Jeff. About your family." Cate shook her head and winced. Meg put a sugarcoated doughnut on Cate's plate. "Here. Try some comfort food."

Cate stared at it and took a bite. She took a sip of black coffee and a bigger bite and rolled a mound of pasty sweetness around her mouth. Bitter and sweet. It made her mouth and nose tingle and tasted good. It pulled Cate into the present.

"Are you with me?" asked Meg.

Cate nodded. "Kayla and Ben. I should be there when they get home from school."

"I took care of that, pending your agreement, because you might be needed here." Meg had called Scott from the ER while she waited for Cate and asked him to pick up Cate's kids and theirs and bring them to Cate and Jeff's house. She also asked Scott to tell Kayla and Ben that Jeff had an accident, that Cate was keeping him company at the hospital, and to call Meg from the car as soon as they were in the car. "That way, the kids can be with friends and an adult they trust, and I can stay with you, and if the timing feels right, you can talk to Kayla and Ben. If any of that's not okay, I can still call Scott and change plans."

"Thanks. It's a good plan. Except I don't know what to say to the kids."

"You're a mom. You'll know." At Meg's suggestion, Cate called the school to tell them that Scott would pick up the children. It felt good to do something. Meg asked Cate what else she was worried about.

"I don't know what this will do to my family."

"Of course. You were worried about your family before the accident."

"That's what I mean. Jeff and I had a fight last night. Then we talked this morning, and it felt like we had a chance, we were supposed to talk more tonight. Now ..." Cate's voice cracked. She covered her face and sobbed.

"Oh, Cate!" Meg wrapped her arms around Cate's shoulders and held her close. "You know I'm here for you."

"I know." Cate cried until she felt relief, then wiped her eyes and sat erect. "I have to pull myself together, enough to call Jeff's parents."

"I'd be glad to call them for you."

"They should hear it from me." Meg suggested waiting until after surgery, after she met with the doctors. Cate thought Karen and Dan would want to come to the hospital from Northfield, an hour south, and decided to call them from the ICU lounge upstairs. While she finished the doughnut and coffee, clearing her head, Meg told her that Indra would bring dinner for everyone to Cate's house that evening. For the next few weeks, Meg would mobilize friends to help with meals and chores and arrange play dates to keep the kids busy.

"What else is pressing?" asked Meg.

"The symposium in six weeks and my class. Jennifer can handle symposium busywork. I posted my PowerPoint, so anyone can cover my class."

While Cate went to the restroom, Meg called Jennifer.

"How did it go?"

"She'll get it done. I told her Jeff's in surgery and why. Hope that's okay. Everyone in the department is thinking about you and Jeff."

"It's fine."

They bused their trays and headed for the ICU.

Upstairs, the ICU receptionist checked a list and reported that Jeff was still in the recovery room, that a note said the doctors wanted to observe him for a while longer before releasing him to the ICU. Unsure what that meant, Cate tramped with Meg to the lounge, where she retrieved her phone and stared at Karen and Dan's home number.

"All you have to do is dial and start talking," said Meg. "It will come." Meg stepped into the hall and returned with a cup of water. Cate sipped and swirled the water around her mouth, savoring the coolness, before she pressed the numbers.

Jeff's mother answered on the first ring. Cate managed to avoid a stammer and glanced at Meg, who nodded encouragement. "I don't know how to tell you this," she said, "but Jeff had a car accident and we're at HCMC, waiting in the ICU lounge for Jeff to arrive and to talk to the doctors. He needed surgery."

"Surgery? For what?" asked Karen. Cate could hear the shock in her voice.

"They had to remove a blood clot on his brain." Cate summarized the events and his condition.

Karen said that she and Dan would leave for HCMC as soon as she reached Dan, who had gone to the grocery store. She was doing administrative work at home that morning and would cancel her afternoon appointments. Dan would likely call with questions as soon as they were on the road.

"You're welcome to use our guestroom."

"Good idea. I'll toss some clothes in a suitcase." Karen offered to call Paul, Jeff's younger brother, and Copper, Cate's younger sister, to let them know what happened. Cate thanked her.

Cate thought about Jeff's parents. Karen, director of Student Health and Counseling at Carleton College, would be a warm and welcome presence. Dan, a retired internist and adjunct professor at the University of Minnesota Medical School, would help all of them understand the nature and seriousness of Jeff's injury. Fifteen minutes later, he called, and Cate related every detail she could recollect. She ended the call, feeling spent.

Cate had to move the car from the ER parking lot to the ramp and returned twenty minutes later, shivering, holding the computer that connected her to work, which felt like the only stable part of her life. She decided to call her office. The department receptionist told her that she had spread the word about Jeff's accident, that everyone wanted to help, from shoveling snow to household chores, that Jennifer would teach her classes, and wanted to assure her that the symposium was on track.

With nothing to distract her, Cate thought about Jeff in the stabilization room. She described to Meg the eerie light that illuminated Jeff from above and made the people in blue and green scrubs look iridescent. "Sounds like a spaceship," said Meg, which elicited a fleeting smile. Cate decided, almost desperately, to see if meditation would quell her anxiety. She concentrated on breathing and watched her thoughts, trying not to give them any energy, as she focused on the maroon metallic chairs, the only objects in the ICU lounge room that had color. Even the pictures were drab. Maroon ... warm not garish hospital maroon ... trying to be cheerful maroon ...

As her racing mind began to slow, the sound of approaching footsteps slipped through the trance. Cate turned to see Jeff's parents in the doorway, their faces painted with worry, and rushed to greet them, just as the ICU receptionist peeked in to say Jeff was leaving the recovery room and the doctors would meet with them soon. Karen and Dan embraced Cate and greeted Meg. "How are you holding up?" asked Karen.

Before Cate could respond, Dr. Watkins and his resident entered, wearing hopeful smiles. Because there was more swelling than expected, they had observed Jeff in the operating room and then the recovery room, considering whether to remove a section of skull to create what they called a window, brain covered only by scalp, but fortunately, the pressure stayed down, and that proved unnecessary. The tube through Jeff's brain would suffice for quick removal of spinal fluid if necessary.

"When will he wake up?" asked Cate.

"We'll continue sedation, the induced coma, for a few days to rest Jeff's brain, then gradually reduce the medication and allow him to wake slowly," said Dr. Watkins. He encouraged questions, but there were none, even from Dan, whose face was bloodless. "You can see him in a few minutes; the ICU nurse will come get you."

Before departing, Dr. Watkins introduced Olivia Carr, the neurosurgery nurse practitioner. Olivia said that neurosurgery would manage Jeff's brain injury, and the critical care team would manage everything else. Olivia—tall, in a white coat over green scrubs—had the bearing of a person comfortable in her role, with a face that radiated calm, a rock-steady handshake, and a voice of kind authority. Cate trusted her at once.

"Let's start with the immediate plan," said Olivia. "We're in the acute phase of care, and our first job is to protect Jeff's brain from further damage, like controlling the pressure and making sure the brain gets enough oxygen." She predicted that they would understand more and have questions once Jamar, Jeff's ICU nurse, showed them all the monitors and equipment in his room and reaffirmed that they could see Jeff as soon as he was stable in the ICU.

"I know acute care is stressful, and I'm sure you're feeling overwhelmed. But I want to say a word about the long haul because TBI recovery takes time. We've learned that families do best when they know that up front," said Olivia.

Cate locked arms with Meg as Dan and Karen stood close.

"It's important to conserve energy from the beginning." Olivia suggested that Cate change her cell phone message, talk only with essential people, use CaringBridge to communicate with friends and family, and choose a friend or relative to keep it current. "One thing you'll hear a lot is that recovery from TBI is a marathon, not a sprint."

I've heard that cliché for everything from investing to navigating life, thought Cate.

"With the kind of TBI Jeff has, we're looking at months of recovery, or more, and marathon is a good touchstone."

Cate closed her eyes and sighed. *It's not a cliché if you're living it*, she thought.

"But he will recover, won't he?" asked Karen.

"That's what we aim for." She asked Cate what she knew about TBIs.

"A little. From news articles about sports and war injuries."

"Then maybe you know there can be long-term problems from TBI," said Olivia.

"You said months or more? What kind of injury does Jeff have?"

"The main problem is torn nerve fibers. You'll learn more about what that means, but let's first get him out of danger." She agreed with Dr. O'Reilly that every brain injury heals differently and that language difficulty, if it occurred, would heal like a stroke. It was too early to predict the degree or pace of Jeff's recovery. She promised that HCMC's experienced team would work as hard as possible to help Jeff reach full recovery, but she could make no guarantees. They would learn more about Jeff, about *his* condition, in the next week as he awakened, then more over the ensuing weeks and months. Olivia paused to let this information settle. Dan, quiet, seemed to understand all of this. Meg mustered a question.

"When Jeff starts to wake up, what will you look for?"

"Basic things that most people take for granted," said Olivia. "Can Jeff say his own name? Does he recognize his wife and parents? Does he know he's in the hospital? Can he speak and understand others? Can he move his arms and legs?"

"Basic? You weren't kidding," said Cate.

"We'll provide lots of information and support. Our first job is to get Jeff safely through the acute phase of care." Olivia answered a few more questions, mainly from Dan, and left with an encouraging smile.

Cate turned to Jeff's dad. "Dan, what's your experience with TBI?" asked Cate.

"None with acute care, but everything they say makes sense. Long term, I can think of two accident patients and one with an injury in Iraq." Dan knew that the vast majority of brain injuries come from accidents, although sports and war injuries garnered the most press and were commonly in the news.

"Are they back to normal?" asked Cate.

"Close. They're close to normal." He faltered, dabbed at his eyes with a tissue, and his voice shook. "Olivia's right. We have to take it one step at a time."

Cate struggled to remain calm as they sat with their thoughts. Meg volunteered to keep CaringBridge up to date. Karen told Meg that Jeff's brother and Cate's sister wanted to visit whenever they could be the most help.

Shortly, a man wearing scrubs, a teal stethoscope wrapped around his neck, introduced himself as Jamar, Jeff's nurse. Cate identified herself and introduced the others. "Have any of you seen Jeff since the accident?" he said. A disarming smile softened his businesslike manner.

"I did. Briefly, in the stabilization room," said Cate.

"You'll find the ICU a lot less hectic. It helps if I tell you in advance what Jeff looks like." They'd find him asleep, hooked up to lots of tubes and monitors, breathing with a respirator through a tube in his mouth, with a large bandage on his head and bruises on his face and body. "Like TV, except that it's Jeff."

Following Jamar, Cate and the others stepped into the hospital chamber, eerily quiet despite monitor chirps and respirator hisses, Jeff motionless and waxen as if in funereal repose. Only his chest moved, expanding passively each time the respirator hissed, then silently contracting. His face was bruised, red and purple.

Cate turned to Jamar. "Where can I touch him?"

"Anywhere there isn't a tube. Go ahead, touch is important for both of you."

While Cate moved cautiously to Jeff's side and touched his arm, Dan, his face drawn and ashen, strode toward Jeff's bed, inspected his son from every angle, and examined each machine and tube.

"You seem to know your way around," said Jamar. "Are you a physician?"

"Yes, but it doesn't help."

"When it's family, everyone's in the same boat," said Karen as she hastened to Dan's side.

Jamar encouraged Cate. "Go ahead, touch him, speak to him too. Familiar voices soothe."

"Will he know it's me?"

"Probably not until he starts to wake up, but it won't hurt and might help." Cate reached for Jeff's hand. It felt flaccid, yet warm and alive. She kissed his bandaged forehead above his bruised left eye, then the corner of his slack lips, avoiding the tube that jutted from his mouth, and put her lips against his ear.

"I love you; I love you very much," Cate whispered.

She lifted the sheet and ran her hand along Jeff's sinewy physique, avoiding his swollen and bruised left hip, caressing the huge scar where a ski had penetrated the front of his left shoulder many years ago. Sleeves encased his legs and inflated with a wheeze every couple of minutes; Jamar said they kept clots from forming in his legs. Cate caressed both cheeks, gently where bruises glared, rested her hand on his chest that expanded as the respirator hissed, surveyed the IV pump and EKG tracing, and stared with horror at two large red tubes that emerged from beneath a sheet in the area of his right groin and seemed to pass through a pump on a table next to the bed. Jamar, anticipating her question, said that it was blood circulating from a large artery through a cooling device and back into a large vein, a protection against fever that would accelerate brain metabolism at a time when his brain needs to remain cool and rested.

"It's not as scary when you know what these things do," said Jamar. He pointed to a tube that emerged from beneath the bandage on Jeff's head and connected to a monitor with dials that indicated brain temperature, pressure, and the amount of oxygen reaching the brain. Cate found the technology strangely reassuring.

"He's so still," she observed. "Even when he sleeps, I can usually sense his energy."

"In a week or less, these tubes will be out," said Jamar, "and he'll be sitting in a chair."

Cate kissed Jeff's ear and whispered again. "I love you, honey. Kayla and Ben love you. Hurry up and get better."

Then it was Dan's turn at Jeff's ear. Cate watched them, father and son, and thought about Jeff and their children.

"You're very pale, Cate," said Karen. "Are you all right?"

"I need a few minutes." Cate escaped to the hallway and sat with her head bent toward the floor, feeling faint. Meg followed and rubbed Cate's back until she sat up. Cate paced for several minutes, glad to move. Then they all trudged to the ICU lounge, where Cate folded her body into a chair. Her eyes rested once again on the textured fabric and metallic arms of the chairs that filled the lounge, entirely maroon, and once again she meditated. *Maroon ... meant-to-be-comfortable, trying-to-be-cheerful hospital maroon ... Cimarron–a castaway ... marooned.*

Cate sat with Meg and Jeff's parents in the lounge, thinking of Jeff marooned, trapped in an inaccessible space, trying not to dwell on her own sense of abandonment. Waiting for the parade to continue. Waiting to meet the critical care physician.

Dr. Rita Menendez and her team of residents and medical students, all in lab coats, swept into the lounge like a bank of white swans.

She was a short, energetic woman with an infectious smile, and she explained that she looked after Jeff's general health and all the injuries except his TBI. She checked them off, fractures and bruises of face, ribs, and pelvis, the collapsed lung, and other bruises around his body. She emphasized that all of them would heal with time. The eye doctors had examined him once more in the operating room and confirmed that the eye itself was not injured. Jeff's heart and lungs functioned well as the respirator did the work of breathing and the suction machine pulled air from the chest tube to keep his lungs expanded. "It helps that Jeff is strong and healthy. Any questions?"

"That tube connected to the suction machine. Will it hurt him?"

"No. It goes to a space outside his lungs, not into them."

"I guess that's good," said Cate in a thin voice. There were no more questions, Dr. Menendez smiled, and the swans left. Cate looked at Dan.

"I think Jeff's in good hands. Everything I see and hear makes sense."

Cate, needing to move again, walked to the end of the hall, to a window where bundles of yellow light mottled the snow-covered ground. Karen joined her, and they stood shoulder to shoulder. "It's so hard to see Jeff like that," said Karen.

"Harrowing," said Cate.

"We'd like to stay close, to be with Jeff, and to help you and the kids. I've taken the week off and can take more, and Dan's completely free except for a few obligations that he can change."

"Having you close will be the most help, especially for the kids. They love you." Cate explained that friends would bring food and help around the house to free time for everyone.

"I might want to do some cooking anyway, even if it's apple pie."

"The kids love your apple pie. We all do."

They hugged, and Cate glanced at her watch, surprised to see that it was half past three, time for Scott to call from the car.

"Are you ready?" asked Meg.

"I'm ready."

They returned to the lounge just as Meg's phone rang. "Hi, Scott; are the kids okay?"

"They're here. Is this a good time?" Meg glanced with raised eyebrows at Cate, who nodded and cleared her throat.

"Put your phone on speaker," said Meg. "I'll do the same."

"Hi, Kayla and Ben," said Cate.

"How's Dad?" asked Kayla, her voice tentative. Ben, in a voice barely audible, echoed his sister.

"Dad's asleep and resting. Like Scott told you, he had a car accident and has to stay in the hospital for a while."

"Is he okay, Mom?" said Ben. "Can I talk to him?"

"He needs to rest, sweetie."

"Does he have a concussion like I did?"

"Yes, an even bigger one than yours. That's why he needs to rest like you did. Grandma and Grandpa are here too. Want to say hi to them?"

"Hi, pumpkins," said Karen. "Grandpa and I are in luck. We get to stay with you for a few days."

"You're staying here?" asked Kayla.

"Yup, if that's okay with you and Ben," said Dan. Both kids expressed delight, their voices stronger.

"Good, we'll see you around dinnertime," said Grandma Karen.

"Hi, Evie and David," said Meg. "Love you. Have fun, and I'll see you soon."

"Love you," said Evie and David in unison.

"Hug Dad for me," said Kayla.

"Me too," said Ben.

"I will. You guys have fun," said Cate.

"Stay as long as you need to," said Scott. "We'll be fine here."

Cate rang off and sank into a chair near the window, holding her head in her hands, thinking about her family, and weeping.

CHAPTER ELEVEN:

That Evening and the Next Morning

Cate thought about her family and her home as her slate-blue Accord crept up the driveway. Home, the place she and Jeff had chosen to have a family, a two-story stuccoed brick structure with tall windows, a mansard roof, a two-car garage, poplars, oaks, and locust trees in a suburban cul-de-sac. She eased into the garage and turned off the engine. On Mondays, Jeff usually beat her home, but his garage space sat empty. Across the void, the remains of perfectly stacked firewood lined the wall, Jeff's handiwork, not a log out of place. They needed to order more, but Jeff did that, and she had no idea whom he called. She gripped the steering wheel to keep from screaming.

Meg waited outside her own car.

Cate checked her watch. Roughly eight hours had passed since the call from HCMC. She pulled down the visor and looked in the mirror, wiped tears from her chin, and plucked lipstick from her open purse, but her fingers trembled too much to use it. She tossed it back and grabbed the purse and her computer.

The children.

She peered again at the mirror, painted her face with a smile, and pushed open the car door. "Do I look okay?"

"Except for the smile." Meg squeezed Cate's shoulder. "Just be yourself, and they'll be fine."

Cate leaned against the car and let the smile fade. Her legs shook as she entered the mudroom, removed her boots and coat, and paused outside the kitchen door. As she twisted the knob, she heard Grandma Karen's voice mention Auggie Pullman and knew she was reading *Wonder.* Once inside the kitchen, with a good view of the porch eating area, she saw the two boys, Ben and his friend David, nestled in Karen's lap on the couch, and Kayla and Evie at the table playing chess with Grandpa as Scott watched. Ben jumped from Karen's lap, knocking *Wonder* to the floor, and ran to hug her. Kayla caught a corner of the chessboard and sent a black rook and a couple of pawns scattering as she ran too. Cate crouched and extended her arms.

"How's Daddy?" asked Ben. He hadn't used Daddy since he was five.

"He was asleep and resting when I left."

"When's he coming home?" asked Ben.

"Soon." Cate's voice trembled. She cleared her throat, steadied her voice, and guessed, "Probably in a couple of weeks."

"That's too long." Ben pushed deeper into her arm.

"It does seem long, but Dad needs time to get better."

"Can't we visit him?" asked Ben. "We can read to him like he does when we're sick."

"In a few days, sweetie," said Cate.

"Let's call him," said Ben.

"I know he'd love to hear your voice, but right now, he needs to sleep."

"We can wake him up and tell him that we love him. Then he'll sleep better."

Kayla gave Ben a big-sister look. "Mom's saying that Dad needs rest to get better."

Cate nodded in agreement.

"Maybe Daddy will dream about us," said Ben, with a sad look.

"Bet he will. I'm gonna dream about him," said Kayla.

"Darn. Daddy was gonna help us make a snowman," said Ben.

"We can still make one," said Kayla. "We can do it together after dinner."

“We sure can,” said Dan. In his hands were the rook and pawns that Kayla had knocked to the floor; he placed them back on the squares where they belonged.

“Let’s make it a snow family,” said Karen. “I can help design it.” Grandma Karen, an amateur sculptor, had once carved the bust of Princess Kay of the Milky Way from a ninety-pound block of butter at the Minnesota State Fair. A picture of Grandma Karen, the buttery bust of Princess Kay, and Jeff, only eight years old and bursting with pride, hung in the family gallery in the back hall.

“It’s a deal—a snow family after dinner,” said Cate. “I still have fruit and vegetables for the face, the hat, and buttons.”

“We can use Dad’s red scarf,” said Kayla.

“And his big hat,” said Ben.

“Nice,” said Cate, stifling tears, as both children watched her, their eyes cautious.

Karen pointed to brown bags on the kitchen counter, and Cate smelled food. Indra had dropped off Chipotle along with brownies and a casserole to freeze. “Bet you’re all hungry,” said Cate. The bags held chips, a big container of guacamole, and trays of barbacoa, chicken, and all the fixings for burritos. Dan and Karen carried the trays to the four-season porch, where they had set the table like Thanksgiving, a bridge table pushed against the porch table, both tables covered with bright blue and orange tablecloths.

From the doorway, Cate’s eyes wandered through the large porch, deceptively festive, filled with family mementos. In one corner sat a two-foot copper and bronze moose with curlicue copper eyes and springs for legs that the boys found at the Gunflint Lodge on a camping vacation to the Boundary Waters. A small brass lion from their South African honeymoon, bold and whimsical, climbed the three-foot Eiffel Tower that Meg and Scott had given them on their first anniversary. Cate had chosen the large coffee table, made of black and white fabric that resembled a Holstein, to celebrate Jeff’s new lab. The room worked.

Kayla and Ben made burritos, and the others followed. Everyone ate quietly. “How was school today?” asked Cate.

"It was fun," said Kayla. Evie, who was in the same sixth-grade class, agreed. They'd used Google Earth on the computer and Google Maps on cell phones to visit places they'd only heard about.

"That's a good way to travel," said Karen.

"And learn geography," said Cate.

"Geography. That's what the teacher called it. We started with our own houses on Google Maps," said Kayla.

"You have to see the picture of our house on Google Maps, Dad." Evie looked at Scott. "It shows you mowing the lawn, and you're not wearing a shirt!"

"Really?" said Scott. "That's a picture I've got to see."

"Me too," said Meg.

Evie opened the app on her phone, showed him the picture, and passed it around. "Nice bod," said Cate. Meg bared her teeth at Cate in a fake growl, and they both laughed.

Kayla and Evie's class had traveled first to England, homed in on London, and found Big Ben and Tower Bridge. The most fun was finding places on Google Earth where kids in the class were born. First, they found Mogadishu on the classroom globe, then on Google Earth; they did the same with Amritsar in the Indian state of Punjab. Once they saw the pictures, they encouraged their classmates to talk about their homelands.

"How about you guys?" asked Cate. Ben and David were classmates in third grade.

"Our class split into two groups and did cool science experiments," said Ben. "I made plastic from vinegar and milk."

"I didn't know you could do that," said Dan.

Ben, sounding professorial, explained the process in detail. He'd made a flat blue disk with a hole in it to use as a keychain. "You know what, I'm gonna put Dad's initials on it and give it to him."

"What a nice idea!" said Dan.

"What about you?" Meg asked David.

"We used real science to study the color wheel. The teacher called it chromatog ... umm ... tography," said David, grinning with enthusiasm. On the ends of paper towel strips, they had painted stripes with magic markers and dipped the ends in water. The purple marker separated into red and blue."

"That sounds like fun," said Scott.

"It was fun. After that, we had to close our eyes, and the teacher did the same thing. From the colors on the strip, we had to guess the color of the magic marker. I saw blue and yellow and knew the marker had to be green."

The conversation continued, lively and distracting. When they finished eating, Karen and Dan resealed the food containers, Meg and Scott cleared the tables with the help of the four kids, and Cate gathered her thoughts.

When she felt ready, Cate led Kayla and Ben into the family room and perched on a cushioned chair in front of the windows. Kayla and Ben faced her on the matching ottoman. "I want to talk about Dad's accident, but I thought I'd start with your questions?"

"How did it happen?" asked Kayla.

"A car coming in the opposite direction hit Dad."

"You mean a head-on collision?" asked Ben, the Quarter Midget driver.

"Yes. The collision totaled Dad's car and sent him to the hospital."

"In an ambulance?" asked Ben.

"That's how people get from accidents to the hospital," said Kayla, with a trace of impatience and a brow furrowed with worry.

"I didn't need an ambulance when I crashed my car," said Ben. "Mom and Dad drove me."

"Dad's accident was worse. A concussion knocked him out."

"Is he still knocked out?" asked Ben. His eyes pleaded for reassurance.

"No. He woke up. Then the doctors gave him medicine to make him sleep, because sleep helps his brain heal, and he's still sleeping." Cate, attentive to their reactions, plunged ahead. "There's more. Dad hit his head on the steering wheel, hard enough to fracture his skull." She pointed to her scalp, just above her left forehead. "The fracture was small, but it tore a vein inside his skull that bled and caused a blood clot, which the doctors had to remove and stop the bleeding."

"You mean Dad had an operation?" asked Kayla.

"That's right. The blood clot is gone."

"My fracture hurt when I broke my arm," said Ben. "Does Dad's skull hurt?

"The medicine that makes him sleep also helps his pain."

Kayla grew quiet and thoughtful. Ben tapped his fingers twice against his knee, paused, and began a steady rhythm of two-taps against his thigh. Cate asked Ben what he was worried about, but he didn't answer.

"Did Dad hurt anything else?" asked Kayla.

Cate told them about Jeff's fractured hip, ribs, and cheekbones but omitted the orbital fracture that would only add worry.

Cate stretched out her arms for hugs, and the children came to her side. Kayla pressed against her and returned the hug, but Ben felt like a rag doll, arms dangling. Cate lifted his chin and gazed at his piercing blue eyes, so much like Jeff's. "Tell me what you're worried about, kiddo," she said.

"Is Dad going to be okay?"

"It may take a while, but I think he will." Cate tightened the hugs. At least she could offer them the safety of her body. Kayla rested her head against her mom, but Ben remained limp. "Honey, what's the matter?"

"I didn't need medicine to sleep. I was awake and you and Daddy stayed with me."

"You didn't stay tired, and Dad won't either."

"Bet he'll dream about us tonight," said Kayla.

Cate shot her a grateful look.

Ben's two-taps slowed, then stopped, and tone returned to Ben's body. Still encircled by Cate's arms, Ben wrapped his arms around his mom and returned the hug.

Neither Kayla nor Ben had more questions. Cate led them back to the kitchen, where decorations for snowmen waited on the island.

"Ready?" asked Karen. Kayla picked up her dad's red scarf and a gray wool hat with a tassel.

"No!" Ben screamed. Cate looked up, alarmed. "I want a better hat." He grabbed the floppy wine-colored fedora, the one Jeff packed for vacations. "And I want the black scarf."

"The hat's okay if you want it that badly," said Kayla, "but we agreed on the red scarf. Red looks good on a snowman."

"The red scarf's okay," said Ben after a moment, and Cate's alarm eased.

"Let's get started, and we can figure out the rest of the clothes later," said Karen, pointing to the coats and leading the way outside.

In the front yard, each of the four children packed snow into fist-sized balls and rolled them in the wet snow. Ben, complaining that David crossed in front of him and used his snow, threw a snowball at David. Scott directed the boys to different parts of the front yard, and Cate reminded Ben that David was his friend, there to keep him company. Ben wouldn't apologize but gradually rolled his snowball closer to David, and the boys shared smiles.

When the balls of snow grew large, the adults pitched in. Grandpa and Scott helped stack the balls, and Grandma Karen directed the family composition, arranging two children in front of two adults, showing the four kids how to fill in gaps between the figures so that the bottoms and torsos of the four figures touched, creating a family unit. The arms of the two adults crossed and met in front, above the heads of the children. Kayla showed the four kids how to position coat buttons so that the torsos turned slightly toward each other.

"This one is Daddy," said Ben. He reached up and placed the floppy fedora on the tallest snowman, and Kayla wrapped the scarf around his neck. Cate handed a carrot to each of the two boys and asked them to look at the buttons and put the nose where it should go. "Hey, you gave David the wrong carrot," said Ben, grabbing the thicker carrot from David and handing him the thin one. "This is Dad's nose."

"It's just a snowman," said David.

"It's my dad," said Ben. "It has to be right."

"Okay," grumbled David.

"Hey, Mom's nose is important too," said Kayla.

The boys stuck the carrots in the middle of the adult heads, pointed slightly toward its mate like the buttons. Next came grape eyes, broccoli ears, red pepper mouths, and green pepper ears. Fresh rosemary hair peeked out from Jeff's gray hat and covered the top of the other adult head above the carrot. Karen showed them how to make the snow family's faces happy.

"Hey, Grandma," said Kayla. "We only have a hat and scarf for Dad. We need more clothes." Karen agreed and dispatched Cate to find garments for the other figures while Karen continued to help the kids shape the snow family.

On the way to the hall closet, Cate glanced out the window at snow Jeff, jaunty in a floppy fedora and red scarf. Suppressing tears, she thought about the real Jeff lying comatose in the ICU. She continued to the back hallway and rummaged through the closet, selecting hats, including the blue bonnet she wore whenever Jeff donned his floppy fedora and several multicolored scarves, before hurrying back outside. The kids loved the blue bonnet for the mom figure and the stovepipe hats from last Halloween for the snow children. Karen showed them how to wrap the scarves, long and flowing, to pull the family together.

"Well, what do you think?" asked Karen.

"Excellent!" declared Kayla as Ben stood quietly, and the rest applauded. Scott snapped a picture of the kids and Cate in front of the snow family with his iPhone, which Kayla said she would bring to Dad so they could all be together like the snow family. Scott took more pictures of the whole group, and Dan took a couple that included Scott, for his family.

Tired and satisfied, the group returned to the porch, where they enjoyed Indra's brownies with milk and coffee.

* * *

The next morning, Cate stood on the front stoop in fleece slippers and a down coat over pajamas as the children waited next to the snow family. When the bus arrived, Kayla and Ben waved from the window until they disappeared around the curve. Cate let her eyes linger on the snow family, a hand against her heart, her eyes moist.

Ben had asked when the snow family would melt.

Back in the kitchen, the smell of scrambled eggs, green peppers, onions, and cheese, one of Grandpa Dan's famous breakfasts, which he usually put together for Sunday brunch in Northfield, whet Cate's appetite. The children had scarfed down every morsel of the first batch, and Dan had started anew while the kids waited outside. Karen handed Cate a hot cup of French roast.

"Hope you slept well," said Cate.

"Your guest room is very comfortable," said Dan.

"Too comfy. We might never leave," said Karen.

"Stay as long as you like. It's a treat for the kids to have you here. For me, too," said Cate.

"Not a good time to be alone," said Karen. "I was able to take a couple weeks off, and then it's winter break, so we can stay until someone else needs the room. I can commute to work from here if it comes to that."

"I didn't have to arrange time off," said Dan.

"Enjoy your retirement quietly," said Karen. She caught Cate's eye and winked.

"You're keeping busy, though," said Cate. "I saw you immersed in Rosetta Stone last night."

"I'm learning Mandarin for our China trip in May," said Dan.

"Impressive."

"Keeps my brain healthy," said Dan. Karen glared at him and rolled her eyes. Dan mouthed an apology and looked away.

"We'll get to the hospital by late morning," said Karen. "Interested in joining us for lunch?"

"Sure. I'm going straight to the hospital, then to the university if I can get away, but I'll be back."

"The university?" asked Karen.

"For an hour. Enough to make sure I'm not leaving anyone in the lurch."

"Then we'll see you shortly. This afternoon, we'll be sure to get home before the kids, so you can stay," said Karen.

"Would you mind defrosting something for dinner?"

"That reminds me," said Karen. "Indra called first thing to say she's arranged a slew of meals for your freezer, and she made eggplant curry for tonight, the recipe your kids like."

"Your kids like eggplant curry?" asked Dan.

"Kayla has adventurous tastes, and Ben will experiment if Kayla cajoles or teases him. If he didn't like to keep up with her, he'd be living on cereal and bananas." Cate excused herself and hurried upstairs.

In the bedroom, Jeff's half of the bed lay undisturbed, a reminder that life had gone off the rails. Yesterday morning, the day had begun with spent anger, with promise and hope.

Cate entered the closet, tossed her pajama top down the laundry chute, listened as it slid to the mudroom below, removed her pajama pants, and listened again. Cate resisted an urge to take every sweater, every shirt, every garment from closet shelves and hangers and toss them one by one down the chute. She snorted at the absurdity, but she and Jeff loved that laundry chute. She pushed on, doing floor exercises to get her body moving, and allowed extra time for the shower massage to pound her body with droplets as hot as she could stand, toweling her skin with vigor. *A laundry chute, exercises, and a shower massage*, thought Cate. *Soothing and predictable.*

She thumbed through sweaters on hangers until she found a taupe wool pullover that Jeff had given her and a skirt that matched. She dressed slowly, trudged down the stairs, kissed Karen and Dan as cheerfully as possible, and headed for the hospital.

CHAPTER TWELVE:

Later that Morning, Hospital Day 2

Cate reached the ICU, pushed a chair next to Jeff's sleeping form, and tried to relax. But the respirator hissed, Jeff's chest expanded and contracted, and Cate's emotions swung like a pendulum out of control. At one end, a whirlwind of thought and emotion too powerful to process. At the other, emptiness and numbness. She couldn't sit still and decided to try a walking meditation, found a quiet corridor not far from the ICU, and walked until the pendulum swings subsided.

Back in Jeff's room, she lay her head on his shoulder, her head lifting slightly with each respirator-driven expansion of his chest, her arm extended along his, fingers on his wrist, feeling his steady pulse. She raised her head to inspect the tubes that sprouted from his bandaged scalp, the stain of Betadine that browned the gauze and smelled like iodine, the machines that monitored and supported his comatose life. She let her head fall again to his shoulder, fused to his breath and to his pulse, and fell into a shallow sleep.

* * *

HCMC provided a PowerPoint presentation for families every Thursday morning, still two days away, and a Consumer Guide, both courtesy of the Minnesota Brain Injury Alliance. Olivia had left the guide, and Cate awoke to find Meg reading it. "Hi, Meg. When did you get here?"

"A few minutes ago. How was your nap?"

Cate sat up and stretched her cramped neck. "Restless, but I needed it."

"This guide," Meg held it up, "has a two-page summary of TBI symptoms. Up for hearing about it?"

"I'll settle for a beating heart."

Jamar entered and pressed the bell of his stethoscope against Jeff's chest, teal tubes joined to human ears. He scanned the monitors and, with a grin, said they were all happy. Earlier this morning, Jeff had tried to fight the respirator, a good sign that meant his brain was working, although it prompted an extra dose of medication. Cate's eyes followed Jamar out the door. In the hallway, a patient on a gurney rolled toward an uncertain destination. Cate and Meg walked to the lobby café, returned with lattes, and watched Jeff sleep.

Cate checked the time on her iPhone. "Darn it, it's too late. I wanted to spend an hour at the university before lunch with Karen and Dan in the cafeteria," said Cate.

"You're too conscientious."

"A lot of people depend on me. I'm used to being reliable."

"The phone is reliable."

"Not good enough. Maybe I can get away this afternoon."

Around eleven, Karen and Dan arrived. Dan marched around the room, checked the monitors, looked at all the tubes, and felt Jeff's pulse. "Everything looks good," he said as he slumped into a chair next to Karen.

"Is it easier when you play doctor?" said Karen, thumping his shoulder, trying to smile.

"It makes me feel a little less useless. He's our son, and there's not a goddamn thing I can do to help." Tears ran down his cheeks.

"Sorry, honey. I was teasing, but it wasn't funny." Karen placed a protective arm around Dan, who sighed and rested a hand on hers.

"Dan, maybe you can help Jeff by helping me," said Cate. "Is he in the best place, getting the care he needs?" Dan surveyed the room, gathering his thoughts.

"I think so. Even though this isn't my field, I like what I see, and HCMC has an excellent reputation."

"Thanks. I'm glad you're here for Jeff, for me and the children."

"It's a good time for the kids to have a grandfather," said Karen.

"A grandmother too. The kids need both of you. And so do I."

Cate's eyes moistened as she thought about her own parents, gone before the kids were born. Kayla and Ben would've loved Grandma Midge. Grandpa James, on the other hand, might have disappointed them, as he had Cate. Throughout her childhood, he'd been misanthropic, a liquor salesman who sometimes claimed to work when he had no job, a father both present and absent who showed no empathy for Cate when Sally died. Grandma Midge kept the peace, ran the household, sold cosmetics at a department store, and dressed with style and taste despite limited funds, attributes she passed to Cate, whom she encouraged. Cate studied violin and played well enough in high school to perform with the Washington University Orchestra when they needed extra strings, a proficiency, along with excellent grades, evidence of leadership, and a thoughtful essay, that earned Cate a scholarship to the University of Pennsylvania.

After Cate started college, her mom divorced, and two years later remarried. Her stepfather, Otis, owned three McDonald's; suddenly, there was money for a summer trip to Europe after her sophomore year and a junior year in Aix-en-Provence. Otis, a strong and generous man, was a good father to Cate and would've been a good grandfather, but he, too, died before Kayla and Ben arrived.

"You look far away," said Karen.

"I was thinking about my parents and sister and my stepdad."

"Midge and Otis were lovely people," said Karen. Grandpa James had passed well before Cate met Jeff. Less than a year after their wedding, Midge and Otis both died from heart attacks—Midge first, Otis two months later.

"While you were thinking about your family, I was admiring your pictures," said Karen. She pointed to the photographs Cate had taped to Jeff's wall. Kayla and Ben in a field of spring tulips, the children playing Roughhouse with Jeff while Cate watched, all four of them on an ocean beach in Cape Cod. They talked of happier times, but for Cate, the heaviness persisted.

After lunch, Karen and Dan left to do errands. Meg, the only person who knew about Cate's marital misgivings, remained, and Cate wanted to talk. She and Meg walked from Jeff's room to the lounge, where Cate described the encounter the night before the accident and the hope of reconciliation the next morning. "It feels like Jeff's accident was my fault. Like it wouldn't have happened if we hadn't fought."

"Cate, there's no way you're responsible for Jeff's accident."

"My sister Sally died because we fought."

"Sisters have arguments. You yelled at her, you chased her, but you didn't chase her into the street. You certainly didn't chase Jeff onto the highway."

"It feels like I did."

"I've had that feeling too, remember? When my sister was depressed, all I did was scold her for not doing her schoolwork and making our parents worry. I did nothing to help her."

"Meg, you didn't make Ellie suicide."

"Exactly. That's what you told me at the time."

Meg's younger sister, a high school junior, had overdosed early in their sophomore year at Penn. When Meg returned from the funeral, behind in her work, unable to concentrate, worried about her parents, isolating in her room, Cate gathered friends and force-marched Meg to student health. She made Meg talk about her sister and her loss. That was when Cate told Meg about Sally and her childhood nightmares.

Shared loss deepened their friendship.

"Shit. Too many worries and too much guilt," said Cate. She reached for Meg's hand and held it. "Thanks, I'm not sure what I would do without you."

"Hey, it's a long friendship. We take turns."

CHAPTER THIRTEEN:

Tuesday Afternoon, Hospital Day 2

That afternoon, Cate spent thirty minutes hidden in Jennifer's University office, discussing symposium details and the class Jen was covering. When she returned to her office, a steady stream of well-wishers interrupted, knocking even when she closed her office door. Her graduate students had no urgent questions, her class was covered, her projects were on track, and she had no pressing reason to be there. Yet she found her office comfortable and secure. She opened her computer and worked on a nonurgent journal article, even though it felt selfish to be there. After another hour, her discomfort grew. She slung her computer bag over her shoulder and returned to HCMC to sit with sleeping Jeff.

Amid respirator hisses and monitor chirps, she opened the computer to address mindless busywork not completed at the university. Her email had filled with notes from well-wishers. Thinking of Olivia's advice, she set the out-of-office reply to thank people for their concern and direct them to CaringBridge. She closed her computer, thrust it aside, and moved her chair next to Jeff. She kissed his forehead, held his warm and flaccid hand, and felt his reassuring pulse, absorbing its energy, feeling his vitality spread from her fingers along her arm to her heart, joining his heart to hers.

In the late afternoon, Karen called to suggest a restaurant excursion because the kids were restless. It was Asia week at the children's school, so Cate thought of Big Bowl, a family favorite. Cate was the last to arrive for dinner. She found everyone engaged, talking and laughing. They'd already ordered.

The food arrived family style, slippery chow fun noodles with chicken, kung pao beef, sesame peanut noodles, and pad thai with shrimp, Cate's favorite, which Kayla made sure to include. Dan had ordered lettuce wraps and showed the kids how to spread hoisin sauce on the lettuce, add chicken and crispy rice noodles, wrap, and munch. "They're yummy, Grandpa," said Ben.

"How's Dad?" asked Kayla. Ben looked up sharply and started a rhythm of two-taps.

"Good, but still sleeping," said Cate.

"I want to visit," said Kayla. "Soon."

"I promise we won't wake him," said Ben. Cate took a deep breath and looked at Karen and Dan, who nodded.

"I'm not sure he'll be awake, but tomorrow evening we can visit for a short time, maybe five minutes. Would that be okay?"

"Yes!" said Kayla. Ben's two-taps slowed.

"Did I tell you that Dad has a cool new haircut?" Cate had decided to dispense information gradually, monitoring Kayla and Ben's reactions. "They had to shave half his head."

"Because of the operation?" said Kayla.

"That's right. So his hair didn't get in the way," said Cate.

"He's bald like Grandpa?" asked Ben. "I don't want him to be bald."

"Only one side until it grows back," said Cate.

"I want to see his new haircut," said Kayla. "Now. Before it grows back."

"You might not see it this visit. His head is covered by a big bandage. He looks like a prizefighter because his face is bruised." Cate watched the kids imagine what their dad looked like.

As the dinner drew to a close, Kayla, who'd taken charge of passing food, grew quiet. Ben clung to Cate, although his two-taps had stopped. He rode home with his mom, and Kayla accompanied the grandparents.

Once at home, settled in the family room, Kayla eyed the empty space on the couch where Jeff usually sat reading the newspaper or something related to work. "I wish Dad was here and not in the hospital," she said, staring out the dark window.

"Me too," said Ben.

"We all do," said Cate.

Dan opened the hearth and invited the children to help light a fire. Karen asked about school.

"We're learning about Asia," said Ben. His teacher used a Chinese yo-yo, spinning on a string between two sticks, to talk about balance and gravity. Kayla had studied natural disasters in China during the past year—July floods, a September earthquake, an October landslide—and had organized her class to collect money for UNICEF.

"Mom, will Dad be home by Christmas?" asked Kayla.

"I talked with the doctors about that this morning," said Cate. "Dad's probably going to need the hospital for several weeks, but he might come home for a visit on Christmas Day. It's too early to know." Ben's eyes widened, and Kayla looked worried. "Whether or not he visits on Christmas, sometime after that, he'll come home for good."

Dan waited for Cate's information to sink in, then invited the kids to add logs to the fire. The activity, the crackling warmth, and the dancing flames helped, and Grandma Karen brought cups of hot chocolate. Both kids lowered their heads into books, sipping and reading until bedtime.

Shortly after lights out, Cate pressed her ear against Kayla's door. Silence. She opened open the door a crack, peeked in, and watched her sleep. Cate closed the door, stepped across the hall to Ben's room, and listened again. More silence. The door squeaked as she turned the knob. *I have to get Jeff to fix that.* She shook her shoulders to chase away the thought, looked in, but did not see Ben. She switched on the light; his bed lay empty. She returned to Kayla's room and discovered Ben in the top bunk, an arm reaching downward toward his sister, who slept on the outside of the bed, close to the edge and to her brother's arm. Cate thought of Jeff. He would have stood with Cate, pressed against her, holding her hand, enjoying the tenderness that the children showed to one another.

Cate descended to the kitchen, made a cup of tea, trudged to the peninsular porch, and set her cup on the glass table. While Karen and Dan remained in the family room, Cate gazed through the windows at the floodlit blue spruce and the yews grayed by winter, which rose from the snow like statues planted in white earth.

CHAPTER FOURTEEN:

Wednesday, Hospital Day 3

Cate tramped into Jeff's room hoping for signs of alertness but found him waxen and still. The same lifeless droids monitored the inner workings of Jeff's body and traced his heart as the respirator hissed and his chest yielded to its pressure. Gently, Cate kissed his full lips, his chiseled cheekbones distorted by bruises, thought about his blue eyes hidden behind swollen eyelids, and placed her lips against his ear. "Jeff, it's Cate. I love you. Kayla and Ben love you too. They're going to visit you tonight." Jeff didn't stir. Cate sank into the vinyl armchair next to the bed and rested her arm on his. She closed her eyes and, for several minutes, lingered on the threshold of consciousness, neither asleep nor awake, until she fell into a brief and fitful slumber. When she woke, she was surprised to feel aroused, remembering Jeff's arms wrapped tightly around her, his body suspended above her, wondering if they would ever have that again.

* * *

Later that morning, as Cate sat reading an article in the *Harvard Business Review,* Olivia stopped by to say they'd begun to taper sedation. If all went well, Jeff would wake up free of agitation, and they could remove the respirator and most of the tubes. By Monday, perhaps this weekend, he'd leave the ICU for a surgery floor.

As Olivia departed, Cate tried to visualize Jeff sitting in the chair, chatting and smiling, although she knew that was more than Olivia had promised. This evening, when the kids visited, he'd still be asleep, breathing with a machine, guarded by monitors. It might be better to wait until he was off the respirator and alert, but the kids needed to see him. She knew Kayla could handle it, but she worried about Ben's anxiety.

Even before Jeff's accident, Ben would wear nothing but navy-blue fleece pants and a matching hoodie, preferring the oldest and most worn of several identical outfits. Cate knew that eight-year-old boys preferred soft pants and liked to wear the same outfit every day, but since Jeff's accident, his rigidity had become almost frantic. He arranged his room in perfect order and his two-taps at times seemed constant. Karen believed his nervous tics might go away in time; she suggested that Cate push Ben gently through his anxiety, not always yield to it. That morning, Cate had tried. "Your favorite clothes are dirty, honey. I picked out your yellow and black waffle tee and your black joggers. You like those too."

"But I only have one set. I'd wear them if I had two."

"Really? Why two?"

"I don't know. It feels better." Ben wouldn't dress until Cate extracted his favorite outfits from the dirty laundry and promised to wash them after school, but he did wear the clothes Cate had selected. Cate thought about him in his waffle tee and about Kayla, a lot more flexible, in skinny jeans and her favorite logo top, and wondered how they were doing at school. Cate had spoken briefly with Bonnie, the guidance counselor, and knew she would call if the teachers noticed problems.

Cate would make it as easy as possible, but they had to see their dad. She'd have to trust their resilience.

* * *

She walked into Jeff's room with an arm wrapped around each child, holding them firmly against her.

"See, Dad's asleep and resting." Kayla escaped Cate's arm and walked to her dad. "Go ahead, honey. Touch his arm. Talk to him." Tentatively, Kayla gripped his arm.

"Hi, Dad. I hope you wake up soon."

"It's okay to kiss his cheek," said Cate. Kayla leaned over the edge of the bed and kissed him.

"I love you, Dad."

Ben held back, pressed against his mother. With a reassuring arm around his shoulder, Cate approached Jeff's bed. She took Ben's hand and pressed it against his dad's arm. "See, his arm is warm, sweetie. Say hi to him."

"He can't hear me."

"Maybe he can."

"He can't. He's asleep. And he's all bandaged up."

"The bandage doesn't cover his ears," said Kayla. "I'll bet he hears us."

Ben took in a deep breath and exhaled. "Hi, Daddy," he said, his voice a whisper. "I want you to get better, Daddy." His voice grew louder. "Please get better, Daddy. Please."

"That's good, Ben," said Cate.

"Give him a kiss, like I did," said Kayla.

Ben kissed his dad's arm. Cate lifted him so he could reach his cheek.

They stood there for a few minutes, each of the kids touching their dad, Cate reaching past the children, their backs against her, to touch him too.

They stood together like the snow family.

CHAPTER FIFTEEN:

Thursday, Hospital Day 4

Seventy-two hours after Jeff's admission, his physicians planned to accelerate the sedation taper. "We think he's asleep from sedation, not his injury, but we have to stop the medication to confirm that," said Olivia. They would also remove the monitor beneath Jeff's skull and the thin tube that passed through his brain to the fluid-filled ventricles.

"Is that another operation?" asked Cate.

"No," said Olivia. "They take them out here, in the room." The blood-filled tubes that joined Jeff's groin to the cooling device and all the other devices would also go. Only the IV and the chest tube would remain.

Cate surveyed the respirator and monitors—she had come to trust their magic—and her eyes creased with worry. "Are you sure he doesn't need all this?"

"Once he's more alert and stable, he won't need any of it," said Olivia.

Cate swallowed hard and reached for optimism.

* * *

At ten thirty, arm in arm with Meg, accompanied by Karen and Dan, Cate stepped into the conference room to hear the weekly talk about traumatic brain injury and stroke that families found helpful. Eight anxious faces greeted them; one had a look of terror. Cate slipped into crisis mode, ready to process information, her mind detached and working, her heart burning.

The room darkened, and the presenter, a tall woman with a friendly demeanor, stood calmly at the podium. Cate leaned forward and focused on the part about TBI. The first portion surprised her: Falls caused nearly half of TBIs. Accidents caused the majority of the rest. Sports and war injuries, often in the news, were far less common. She learned that roughly 2.5 million TBI accident patients visit emergency rooms in the United States each year. Although 85 percent have mild TBIs and recover completely, 5.3 million Americans live with permanent TBI disability.

"Wow, I had no idea TBIs were that common," Meg whispered.

Cate's distress increased as the presenter showed MRI and CT images that resembled Jeff's, followed by a list of TBI symptoms that might persist, especially with torn nerve fibers, what she called Diffuse Axonal Injury—loss of memory, moodiness, apathy, irritability or aggression, poor judgment, and lack of insight. Other injuries—such as language problems or visual-spatial skills important for navigating around a house or driving through a neighborhood—occurred with focal injuries to specific parts of the left or right side of the brain, resembled a stroke, and improved over the first few months. But they, too, might not resolve completely. Her anguish didn't ease when the presenter moved to brain injury assessment and rehabilitation tools. Once again, she heard that injury severity or brain imaging does not always predict symptoms or prognosis. Recovery may take many months, sometimes a year or two, with the most improvement in the early months.

Cate, with Meg on one side and Karen and Dan on the other, walked silently to the coffee shop. They sat, sipping lattes. "Well, that was exhausting," said Karen.

"It's good information," said Dan. "Hard to hear, but thorough."

"I thought it was pretty generic, a sketchy roadmap at best," said Meg.

"Yeah, a roadmap for a journey to a vague destination with no timetable," said Cate.

"Won't you get a more specific roadmap about Jeff when we meet with the TBI nurse coordinator?" asked Karen.

"I hope so," said Cate.

"When is it?" asked Meg.

"One thirty."

"Wish I could be there; I have a class to teach."

"I could easily spend a couple of hours at the U, but I'll stay here," said Cate.

"I'm glad you're not pushing yourself," said Karen.

"It's not about pushing. Work is the only place I can lose myself and pretend none of this is real. It's a different journey, where at least I have some control. Sometimes I need that to keep from screaming."

"I understand," said Karen softly. "We certainly can't control anything here except ourselves."

"I think we all feel helpless," said Dan, his voice somber.

"It helps to acknowledge that," said Karen. She pulled Cate close. Dan wiped a tear from his eye.

"It hurts to see Jeff like this," said Meg. She hugged Cate and Jeff's parents and walked slowly out the door, holding her coffee.

"I think I'll call Jennifer at work, for at least a brief escape, to see if there's anything she needs from me," said Cate. She arranged to meet Jeff's parents in the cafeteria at noon or in Jeff's room if she finished the call sooner. They left the coffee shop, and Cate found a remote corner in the lobby.

Jen was one of the few people at work with whom Cate had a social relationship; they went to dinner with spouses. After Cate updated Jennifer about Jeff, they chatted about kids and family before turning to the symposium. A few summaries from symposium speakers and seminar leaders had arrived, clarifying what they would cover. All were satisfactory; one was from Jack Ross.

"Is he back from Japan?"

Cate felt a tension, almost a longing. She missed their talks.

"Yesterday. Preparations for his sabbatical went well."

They chatted for a few more minutes. Jennifer liked filling in for Cate, teaching her class, and said it was more fun for her than work.

She had run her symposium address past Jack and received helpful advice. Something about Jennifer's enthusiasm made Cate uneasy.

After that call, Cate felt an urge to call Jack, whom she hadn't thought about since Jeff's accident. "Hey, good to hear your voice," he said warmly. "How's Jeff?" Cate briefed him about Jeff, the kids, and herself and asked about his trip, which had gone well. He was excited about his sabbatical that would begin in January and last ten weeks. "Remember that Japan is only a phone call away, so let's stay in touch. If I know you, work will keep you centered when everything else is falling apart."

"You do know me. I just said pretty much the same thing about work to Jeff's parents. But I'll miss you."

"I make it sound like I'm about to leave, but I'll be here for another month. If you need to blow off tension with a run in the Fieldhouse, I'm available."

Cate hesitated. She enjoyed those runs and their conversation, but her mind was racing. On Thanksgiving weekend, two weeks before Jeff's accident, Meg had suggested that Cate was getting something from Jack that should come from Jeff, warning that she might be on the way to an affair, which Cate said would never happen. Yet, she had considered what role Jack played in her dissatisfaction with her marriage. After she stopped having nightmares about Sally, before Jeff's accident, twice she dreamed that she was running with Jack on a quiet path through the woods, enjoying the solitude, and had shared a kiss and a passionate embrace. She had awakened aroused and distressed, confused by the sensation of pleasure.

She inhaled deeply to clear her head.

"Wish I had time for a run," she said. I'm barely managing."

"Lunch? You have to eat."

Cate felt lonely and frightened. Something about this conversation felt dangerous.

"Too much to do, so I usually eat at the hospital. But you're right about work. It keeps me centered. I'd like to talk about your plenary address on the second day of the symposium."

"Sure."

"I noticed that part of your plenary overlaps with mine. Would you consider talking more about cultural differences, how Japanese and Western leaders approach globalization differently?" Jack understood the overlap and agreed to revise his plenary.

"Anytime it works for you, give me a call. I'll be thinking about you and your family."

They ended the call, and Cate felt herself relax.

Two pictures rested on her office bookshelf, one of Jeff and her, one of the whole family. The next time she was in her office, she would move them to her desk.

* * *

Jane, the TBI nurse coordinator, greeted Cate and Jeff's parents in the ICU lounge. She wore a turquoise dress that complemented her auburn hair, and she chatted amiably before describing how rehabilitation would unfold. The transfer to inpatient rehabilitation would occur once Jeff could participate in three hours of therapy each day, an insurance requirement.

"I don't get the insurance requirement," said Cate.

"If he's ready for discharge from surgery but can't participate in three hours of therapy, he might need a short stay in a nursing home."

"Are you saying Jeff needs a nursing home?" asked Cate.

"I can't imagine that," said Dan.

"It's unlikely, but it's a possibility I have to mention," said Jane. Prior to transfer, she'd take them on a tour to learn how the components of rehab work together, and when they'd meet Dr. Laura Boulder, the Physical Medicine and Rehabilitation physician who led the team. Dan asked to meet her as soon as possible, and Jane agreed to let her know. After four to six weeks in the hospital, Jeff would continue rehab as an outpatient. Social Service would help with that transition.

"They say he's doing well, waking up before expected, but this morning we heard a lot about TBI symptoms that worry me," said Cate.

"That talk provides important information, but it can be scary. It's likely that Jeff will have some of those symptoms, especially the ones from diffuse axonal injury and some problems with speech from that contusion in the language area. Our goal is recovery, and we work as hard as we can to make that a complete recovery, but we may not get there." Jane paused to let that settle. "What I can promise is support from everyone on our very experienced TBI team, which includes a psychologist to help Jeff and you adjust to whatever develops."

"I hoped for something more definitive about Jeff—what he'll be like, and when he'll recover."

"I wish I could be more definite. Uncertainty is very hard. We'll know a lot more in the next few weeks." Jane smiled. "You're right about him waking up sooner than expected, and that's good news. If you haven't seen him since this morning, you're in for a pleasant surprise."

As Cate entered Jeff's room with his parents, her heart leaped. That morning, Jeff had slept in bed. Now he slept in the recliner. A fresh bandage, much smaller than before, covered his scalp and no tubes protruded from the bandage, his bruised lips, or his groin. The hissing respirator, all the monitors and machines, had disappeared and a thick silence separated Jeff's room from the busy hallway. There remained only the IV and the bubbling chest tube.

Cate hurried to his bedside. "Jeff, it's Cate." His head moved slightly. "Honey, I love you!"

Jamar entered, smiling. "The doctors came right after lunch. You can see their handiwork and he's doing great for hospital day four."

"Day four? He's been here three days."

"In hospital time, day one is the day of admission. Just to confuse you." Jamar smiled.

"Well, they did make the room quieter." Cate could not produce a smile. "How alert has he been?"

"He used his legs to help when we moved him to the chair. He opened his eyes and moved his arms and legs spontaneously, all of which is very positive. We're still tapering sedation. By this afternoon, he should be a lot more alert."

"Has he said anything?"

"An occasional murmur. No words. Try to talk to him."

"Jeff, open your eyes." His swollen eyelids opened and closed. "You understand me!" she said.

"Perhaps. He might be responding to the sound of your voice," said Jamar, "but that's still good." He encouraged Cate to keep talking.

"Honey, you're waking up. You're coming back." His head turned toward her, and his eyes flickered open, unfocused, and closed again. "Kayla and Ben visited. I wish you could remember their kisses."

She sat, stroking his arm, and chatting to him about the kids, about the symposium, about how much she loves him, anything to keep talking. He slept but seemed to breathe more easily. From time to time, his eyes opened, looked in her direction, but did not focus. "Jeff, I know you hear me, and I hope you understand, especially about the kids." His eyes opened, and his head turned as if to search for her. "I'm right here, honey. Your mom and dad are here too." But his eyes closed without making contact.

"It's like stop-and-go traffic," said Jamar. "It moves eventually." Jamar, before he departed, warned that Jeff would remain groggy and wouldn't recognize her, even though her voice soothed him.

"Thanks. One thing I know about myself is that I need information. It helps me cope."

Cate and Jeff's parents continued the chatter. They told Jeff that he'd hurt his head in an accident, was in the hospital and getting better, they were staying in the guest room, and everyone wanted him home.

Eventually, Jeff's parents sought respite in the lounge. Cate sauntered into the hall and retrieved from the vending machine two cans of A&W diet cream soda, the kind Jeff loved and that she rarely drank. Savoring the coldness more than the taste, she meandered back to Jeff's room and held one can against an unbruised portion of his forehead. He stirred. "When you get better, I'll stock the fridge with diet cream."

In late afternoon, Jeff's parents left so the kids wouldn't be alone at home. Scott, Meg's husband, stopped by to visit. He was chatting with Cate when a man knocked on the doorjamb. With an ingratiating smile, the man introduced himself as a representative of the company that insured the driver of the Dodge Challenger. He identified Cate and asked how she was doing. "We'd like you to be comfortable without having to worry about money …"

Scott interrupted. "Exactly why are you here?"

"To provide security and avoid future aggravation."

"If you want to talk, I'm their attorney." He handed the man a business card. "Call me at my office."

"But you haven't heard my offer. It's a good settlement."

"It won't be fair, and it won't be enough. I can tell you it's far too early to talk about a settlement. We haven't a clue what his care will cost. And there's a possibility of disability."

"We're trying to make this easy for Jeff and his family."

"Okay, that's enough. You have my card." The man left, tucking a vinyl case beneath his arm. Scott grimaced and watched the insurance man walk down the hall. "That son-of-a-bitch wants to sweet-talk you into an early settlement."

"I know enough not to sign anything, but I'm glad you were here."

"I shut him down, but you do need an attorney. I can ask a personal injury attorney from my firm to represent you or give you other names."

"Thanks, Scott. Your firm is fine." Cate looked at Jeff and sighed. "Did Meg tell you? If he can't do three hours of rehab, he might need a nursing home."

"There's nothing I can do about that requirement, unfortunately. I wish I could."

"It's been a long, rough day."

"One thing you don't have to worry about is hospital bills. That bastard's insurance company will cover expenses, and if you need financial assistance in the interim, Meg and I would be glad to help. The hospital and his doctors might have to wait to get paid, except for what your insurance pays, but that's common after accidents. At some point, Jeff's health insurer may decide that some of his care isn't medically necessary."

"I'm familiar with prior authorization."

"It won't stop his care. What usually happens is that your attorney writes to the hospital and others to assure them they'll get paid when the claim settles and asks them to continue treatment. The settlement will cover everything his doctors prescribe. If Jeff has disability insurance, his attorney can also help with that."

"He does, and thanks." Scott suggested Keith Williams in his office and offered to bring him up to speed. Cate agreed with thanks and said she'd give him a call. She took a deep breath and surprised herself with a chuckle. "I've never seen that side of you, the tough attorney at work."

"What you saw was a pissed-off friend." Scott grinned. "It's good to see you haven't lost your sense of humor."

"It's in there, somewhere."

"If you're ready to leave, I'll walk you to the car." He touched Jeff's shoulder. "It's Scott, buddy. I'll visit again soon." Jeff didn't respond.

Cate kissed and stroked Jeff's cheek. He made a soft rumble from deep in his throat that she hoped was recognition. She kissed his lips. "I love you, honey." Then she put on her coat and walked with Scott to her car.

CHAPTER SIXTEEN:

Friday, Hospital Day 5

Ben sprinkled his breakfast waffle with maple syrup. Using his knife and fork with precision, he sawed the Eggo into eight equal wedges, carefully placed two fresh blueberries on each wedge, and forked one into his mouth. Kayla looked up, blueberries and syrup dripping from her lower lip. "Just eat the waffle, Ben."

"I am," said Ben. "Mommy, when can we visit Daddy again?"

"When he's not too sleepy or mixed up."

Ben wiped his lips twice, although he'd slipped the waffle into his mouth without touching them. "Tomorrow's the weekend. On TV, people visit on weekends."

"Ben, a weekend is Saturday and Sunday," said Kayla.

"I want to visit Daddy both days," said Ben. "Even if he's sleepy."

"I know you do," said Cate, who'd talked several times to HCMC, Jeff's parents, and Meg about the timing of their next visit. Was it better to see a confused dad who might not recognize them or one who was more like himself? "Not tomorrow, and we'll see about Sunday, but I can't promise."

"Is the bandage smaller? Then we can see his cool haircut," said Kayla. Ben two-tapped twice.

"It's smaller, and yes, you can see his haircut." She reached for her purse, extracted her iPhone, and showed them a picture of Jeff in the recliner. Below the bandage, the left side of his head was shorn of hair. His eyes lacked animation.

"I don't like his haircut, and he looks tired," said Ben, but the two-tapping slowed.

"He looks funny," said Kayla.

"Funny and tired," said Cate with a gentle smile.

"So what if he's sleepy?" said Ben. "We can still visit!"

"The doctors want him to rest, honey," said Cate.

"Hey, was that singing I heard this morning?" said Karen, with a wink at Cate, who mouthed a thank you.

"We were humming, Grandma," said Ben.

"Christmas carols," said Kayla. "It was 'Silent Night.'"

"Grandpa, when are you gonna get us that tree?" said Ben.

"How about this afternoon when you get home?" said Dan. "I made room for it in the family room, see?" The snow leopard chairs in front of the windows had been pushed apart. Beyond the windows, the snow family stood, unmelted.

"We can decorate the tree tonight," said Karen.

"I want Daddy home for Christmas," said Ben. Christmas was two and a half weeks away, but to Cate, it felt like tomorrow.

"Dad might come home for a short visit, but the doctors don't know yet," said Cate.

"Tell Daddy that Grandpa's getting the tree. Then he won't worry," said Ben.

"I'll tell him today," said Cate.

"After it's decorated, I'll take a picture of you guys in front of it," said Dan. "Your mom can tape it to Dad's wall."

"Thanks, Grandpa," said Ben.

The kids donned coats and left. From the family room, the adults watched Kayla and Ben race past the snow family to the bus.

"Thank God they're resilient," said Dan.

"Resilient and scared," said Karen. "Especially Ben."

"I'll call my friend, Bonnie, from the university this morning to check on them. She's the school guidance counselor."

"You have to work?" said Karen.

"Something came up, time-sensitive, about the symposium. I'll make it short."

"You've got a full plate," said Dan. "Would it help if Karen and I finished the Christmas shopping for Jeff and the kids?"

"That's a great idea," said Karen.

"Thanks. I don't know where I'd find the time." Cate choked back tears. What Jeff called *the great Christmas shop* was an annual chore they did together, always managing to surprise each other with purchases made when spousal attention was elsewhere.

Cate lumbered up the stairs and prepared to attack the day. She showered hastily, threw on designer jeans and a brighter-than-she-felt kelly green sweater, and drove to the university. On the way, she called Meg. "I'm surprised you're going to work," said Meg.

"Why does everyone say that? I have to meet with Jennifer."

"You sound irritated."

"That's because I am. Yes, we could probably get it done by phone, but it's easier in person." Her voice faltered. "Meg, it's not irritation. The truth is, I'm scared." Cate choked back tears. "I could end up as the only breadwinner, and I can't jeopardize my job."

"Honey, your job is safe."

"It doesn't feel that way. Nothing feels safe."

"I understand, but Catie, I promise your job will be there."

"When I work, it feels like I'm protecting my family; it's the right thing to do. At the same time, it feels selfish, really selfish, because I love what I do. It's the only sane part of my life, except for the kids, and I'd rather work than watch Jeff sleep." Cate hesitated. "I know I'm feeling sorry for myself. I feel so lost."

"Why wouldn't you?"

"I don't know. It helps to say it."

"Catie, you're overwhelmed and frightened; you're grieving, and you feel guilty if you enjoy something. That's where you are."

"I think that's right."

"Catie, get done what you have to do at work—for heaven's sake, let yourself enjoy it— then go back to the hospital."

Cate felt the heaviness begin to lift. Meg asked about Kayla and Ben. For the rest of the drive, they chatted about kids and school. It felt good to talk about family.

* * *

Light traffic allowed Cate to reach the Nineteenth Avenue parking ramp shortly after eight, forty-five minutes before her meeting with Jennifer. She decided to walk from the West Bank of the campus across the Washington Avenue bridge that spans the Mississippi River to the East Bank, to the elevated path that sits above the Northrop and Coffman quadrangles, a spot that vibrates with student energy, the place to which she gravitated when she needed to recharge.

Standing on the elevated path, Cate sensed the urgency of finals. Students rushed past on bicycles or on foot, and an occasional whiff of hot coffee reached her on the gentle breeze. In the vast Northrop quadrangle, students in multicolored scarves hurried along shoveled paths that outlined and crisscrossed the quad. Clear snow glistened in the afternoon sun and made the scene postcard lovely. She pivoted to look south across Washington Avenue at the quad in front of Coffman Union, crowded as well with scurrying students. She gazed down on Washington Avenue, closed to traffic, populated with busy workers constructing the light rail line that would link the campus with the downtowns of Minneapolis and St. Paul. Everywhere was a sense of purpose. Across Washington Avenue and to the right of Coffman, the broad aluminum sheets of Frank Gehry's Weisman Art Museum glistened in bright sunlight. She removed her gloves and hat to feel the bracing chill of subfreezing temperatures. As she stood there in the center of campus activity, life seemed easier.

Cate descended the stairs and followed the footpath that curved around Weisman toward the pedestrian level of the Washington Avenue Bridge and the path to her office. She eschewed the heated maroon-and-gold structure in the middle and walked along the north side of the bridge that overlooked downtown Minneapolis, enjoying the crisp air against her cheeks and ungloved hands. At the bridge's center, she stopped and gazed at the Mississippi River, almost completely covered with ice.

The Mississippi had fascinated her since her childhood in St. Louis. The river began as a trickle in the Minnesota headwaters at Lake Itasca. A raindrop that fell in the headwaters would flow briefly north, then south through the center of the continental United States, joined by the Ohio, Missouri, and Colorado Rivers and tributaries from thirty-two states, as the river raced larger and stronger past St. Louis and New Orleans, and one hundred miles later merged with ocean waters at the Gulf of Mexico. That trip would take the raindrop ninety days. What would Jeff be like in ninety days?

She'd thought about leaving Jeff. Perhaps he'd found a way to leave her.

As Cate stood on the bridge, she recalled all those hours sitting alone late at night in her home office considering what to do with her marriage, weighing pros and cons, doing nothing while frustration built. It seemed ironic—her most recent journal article, coauthored with Jack—was about conflict resolution.

Jack Ross.

She could talk to Jack. Jack was a delight. Indeed, their conversations had become the catalyst for thoughts of separation.

So much had changed in the tumultuous past week, from the evening confrontation to the morning of the accident, to Jeff's injury and all that followed. She knew, now more than ever, how much she loved Jeff. And how much she loved her family.

She thought about her reverie—the run through the woods with Jack, the imagined embrace—and shivered. She watched the river. She knew she would never leave Jeff. Whatever transpired, the river of her marriage would stay within its banks.

When Cate reached the West Bank, she turned toward her office at the Carlson School of Management. She strode through the large entry hall to the elevators, hoping they were empty. She wanted to face work, not questions.

But the doors opened to reveal Jack Ross. Cate's heart fluttered and sank. "Glad to see you," he said with a friendly hug. "I've been thinking a lot about you and Jeff." His face invited conversation, but he didn't press, which Cate appreciated. She said Jeff was better. "I'm free anytime if you need extra help for the symposium or just want to talk."

"Thanks, Jack," said Cate. "By the way, I appreciate the changes you made to your plenary. It's the perfect launch for the second day." They emerged on the fourth floor. Jack turned right toward the corner office of a respected full professor. She walked to her office opposite the elevator.

As Cate entered, Jennifer rose from her worktable to greet her. Cate would've preferred a few minutes alone, but it was easier to face Jennifer than Jack. "First things first," said Jennifer. "How's Jeff?"

Cate provided a brief update, said she wanted to get back to the hospital as soon as possible, and turned to the symposium file open on the worktable.

"How are you and the kids doing?" asked Jennifer.

"Managing."

"Everyone in the department asks about you."

Cate mentioned CaringBridge. "I want to get through this and back to Jeff."

The urgent symposium issue involved the illness and cancellation of the speaker scheduled to give Sunday's plenary address. They had to agree on a replacement and get it arranged.

"I could give that plenary," said Jennifer. She'd drafted a summary of what she might say, but her subject—the global impact of emerging technology—was already covered in one of the breakout seminars. Jennifer had coauthored an article with Jack on that subject, and the link to Jack irritated Cate.

"We need international speakers, not a panel packed with people from the U of M."

"I disagree."

"Look," said Cate, "if we want to talk about technology, I have an idea." Cate knew a speaker from Oxford University, an expert on the global impact of cloud-based businesses. She pressed the point, and Jennifer reluctantly agreed.

"I want you to know that I'm available if something comes up with Jeff," said Jennifer. "I could give your keynote, even at the last minute. I could also manage your breakout session and make the closing symposium comments for you."

Cate stiffened. "Look, Jennifer, it will be five weeks from the accident. If I need your help, I'll ask. As for the breakout session, I'm going to give Rosie a shot. She deserves that chance, and it'll be easier to supervise than prepare. If you were thinking about someone other than yourself, that might occur to you too."

"Hey, don't rag on me."

"Why not? You deserve it."

Jennifer left, and Cate fumed. She wasn't the only person who could be selfish. It took several minutes for her annoyance to abate.

* * *

When Cate reached the hospital, Jeff was in the recliner, wearing the bright blue terrycloth robe that Cate had bought for him, and the chest tube had disappeared. Sunlight poured through the window and lit his face, still mottled purple with bruises. Although he was half-asleep, the corners of his mouth seemed to edge upward in response to Cate's presence.

Jamar peeked in to say that the medication taper was progressing, and he was doing well, except for a brief episode of agitation with a spike in blood pressure, which would keep him in the ICU for another day of close observation. "Too bad you weren't here an hour ago when he was more alert."

"Has he said anything?"

"A few isolated words that were hard to understand," he said. "His speech will come, and then we can assess how well he can say what he's thinking and what he comprehends. We had him stand and move around, and he seemed to follow instructions, even though he was confused." Jamar offered an encouraging smile and left.

Feeling hopeful, Cate tried to engage Jeff, but he stared without focus at his surroundings. She was still trying when Jane appeared.

"I heard Jeff's coming around."

"I'd like to see more of it myself," said Cate. "Jamar said he's been more alert but still confused. I wish I knew what it's like for him. I'd like to crawl inside his head and see the world as he does."

"It's hard to know what he experiences," said Jane. "He's trying to reassemble a world he once knew from fragments—images, sounds, sensations—and bits of memory that seem vaguely familiar."

"What about emotion?" asked Cate.

"Same thing. Particles of emotion that don't make sense. If there're too many fragments, too much emotion, he gets overwhelmed and agitated. At this point, agitation is kind of a primitive response, like when a baby cries from hunger or a wet diaper but doesn't know why or at least can't tell us. In a way, a healing brain is like a growing brain."

"Primitive in different ways?" Jane nodded, and Cate let that percolate.

"Do you have any questions before I leave?"

"No, but thanks. Information always helps. You've given me a lot to think about."

Shortly after Jane left, Jeff surprised Cate with a glint of life in his eyes. Cate, although hesitant to trust her perception, sensed vitality.

"Ca…t."

"Were you trying to say my name?" said Cate, abandoning caution. The spark lingered for a few seconds and dulled, taking Cate's elation with it. Exasperation filled the void as if Jeff had ignored her with purpose, which she knew couldn't be true.

Cate sank into the chair and rested her head on her hands. Tears blossomed into sobs that made her body shake. She gripped the chair and pressed her back against it, taking solace from the walls, the ceiling, the floor, anything with structure that could contain her. She cried until she felt spent, until uncertainty began to have a structure of its own.

* * *

Perhaps an hour passed before Cate stirred. She thought about a walk outside in the cleansing chill but didn't want to leave Jeff. She looked at him, and his eyes were open, focused.

"Ca…t." This time, Cate knew it was her name. Her heart could tell. Then Jeff was gone again, asleep. Cate kissed his forehead and whispered that she loved him.

She checked her phone and found a text from Rosie asking if it were possible to get together to discuss a thesis question that was blocking her progress, saying she'd understand if Cate could not. Cate arranged to meet her in the hospital lobby, where they found a quiet spot. They resolved the thesis question easily and Cate, with a broad smile, offered Rosie the chance to run Cate's breakout session at the symposium.

"Thank you!" said Rosie. Her freckles glowed with pleasure, the same look that Cate often saw in Mandy, her younger sister and Cate's part-time nanny, whom Rosie had recommended for that position. Cate adored both women.

Mandy, who still helped transport Kayla and Ben to activities and did light housework, had become part of Cate's family. Mandy had requested vacation time to prepare for finals and to work on her senior project, due after winter break, but had called to make herself available when she learned from Rosie about Jeff's accident. Cate was managing with help from family and friends but said she might need more time after winter break, especially when Jeff came home.

Rosie left, and Cate returned to Jeff's room, where a physical therapist was asking him to stand. His eyes were open but cloudy, and he didn't respond to the therapist's voice. She waved her hand, indicating that he should stand. Finally, she gripped his wrist and pulled upward, wrapped a belt around his waist, and guided him out of his room and into the central area of the ICU, then back to the room. He favored his left hip, and his face showed pain, but he followed her instructions. The activity increased his alertness.

"Good job," said the therapist as he settled into the recliner. She smiled at Cate. "Are you his wife?" Cate nodded. "This was his first walk, and he did very well. Jeff, we'll take another stroll this afternoon," she said, and left.

Jeff's eyes fastened on Cate. He stretched an arm toward her and let it fall.

"Hi, sweetie," said Cate. His eyes held neither life nor interest. She sat with him and chatted, a conversation with a silent partner.

* * *

At bedtime, Kayla and Ben chose the book *Jack Stalwart, The Secret of the Sacred Temple: Cambodia,* in which Jack stalwart finds the missing archaeologist who guards the ancient treasure of Angkor Wat. Cate read to them, happy that they'd selected a tale of triumph.

After the story, they lay on their tummies next to each other in Kayla's lower bunk. Cate rubbed their backs, something Kayla had wanted less often as she approached eleven, surprised by the tension in their neck and shoulder muscles. The massages continued until Ben yawned and climbed into the top bunk. Softly, Cate sang "Somewhere Over the Rainbow" and kissed them goodnight.

Downstairs, Dan handed Cate the front page of the *New York Times.* President Obama and Congress were at war with each other, the nation in disarray from tax increases, automatic spending cuts, federal agency layoffs, and postponed education payments to states. For Cate, even bad news was welcome. She read about shoddy mortgage securities and delays producing the Boeing 787—everywhere a dearth of leadership.

Cate put down the *Times,* mounted the stairs, twisted the knob on Kayla's door, and for several minutes watched the children sleep. From the hallway, incandescent light dappled the bed. As Ben lost the last remnant of chubbiness, he resembled Jeff more and more. Kayla, on her side, facing the door, had Jeff's full lips. *Too young to lose their innocence,* she thought.

CHAPTER SEVENTEEN:

Sunday, Hospital Day 7

Mornings began with breakfast, but with a different pace on weekends. It was a routine of normalcy for Cate and the kids, made special by the presence of grandparents. Cate fried lox and eggs, a dish Jeff often made on weekends. He called it Jewish soul food, a recipe he learned from a college roommate.

"These eggs are too runny, Mommy," said Ben, "and the lox is mushy." Yet he kept ferrying food from plate to mouth like an automaton, never touching his lips with the fork.

"Next time, let me make it." Kayla was Jeff's sous-chef.

Cate had deliberately chosen one of Jeff's recipes, and it wasn't working. Grandma Karen cut Ben's toast at his direction into a perfect square without crust, then into four identical triangles, and placed a dab of strawberry jelly in the center of each piece. Kayla licked marmalade from a spoon and reached her spoon toward the jar.

"No double dipping," said Ben.

"What's the big deal? You don't eat marmalade because of the orange peels," said Kayla. "Besides, the jar's practically empty, so you don't have to worry about germs."

"Germs spread." Ben took a careful bite of a triangle, unable to fit the whole triangle into his mouth. Kayla rolled her eyes.

Cate urged them to finish because she had a surprise. “Can you guess what it is?”

“We’re going to visit Dad?” said Kayla. Cate grinned.

“Hooray!” said Ben.

“Yay! I hoped that was the surprise,” said Kayla.

“It’s going to be a short visit, like before. Remember what I told you yesterday? He’s off the ICU and on a regular hospital floor, but he’s still mixed up. Sometimes he doesn’t know who I am, and he may not recognize you.” Ben’s body grew rigid.

“I knew you when I had my concussion,” he said.

“Dad had a bigger concussion, and he had an operation on his head,” said Kayla, although she, too, looked worried.

“If he doesn’t recognize you today, he will next time,” said Cate, taking a risk.

When they reached the hospital, Cate wrapped an arm firmly around each child, as she had before. To everyone’s amazement, they found Jeff walking in the hall, arms draped around the shoulders of two aides, teetering like a battered prizefighter trying to stand after a knockout. He lumbered along, turned, and shuffled back to his room. “Lift your feet when you walk, Jeff,” said the aide who conducted the excursion. He did.

Jeff’s response to verbal instructions thrilled Cate, despite his frailty.

Then he walked past his family with hardly a glance, and her spirits plummeted. She gripped the kids’ shoulders more tightly as the aides eased Jeff into the recliner, waited until he settled, maneuvered the children directly in front of him, and with a free hand, lifted his chin. His eyes found their faces but not their eyes. “Jeff, I brought Kayla and Ben.” His eyes glinted with a spark of life, and his face twitched.

“I think he wants to smile, Mom,” said Kayla.

Cate nodded.

The flash of recognition faded, but the kids had seen it. Jeff’s eyes closed.

“Dad knew you guys, even though he’s worn out from that walk,” said Cate.

"I don't like his haircut," said Ben.

"You saw it already in Mom's picture," said Kayla.

"Yeah, but this isn't a picture," said Ben.

"It's like peach fuzz, Ben. Go ahead and touch the fuzz below the bandage. You won't hurt him," said Cate. Ben started to reach but stopped. Cate took his hand and guided it to Jeff's head. Ben, at first tentative, rubbed his dad's scalp.

"Doesn't it feel like a peach?" asked Cate.

"Like a brush," said Ben. "Hey, Kayla, you try."

Kayla touched her dad's head and smiled. "You're right, Ben. It's like a bristly brush." Cate laughed, and Ben's rigid body relaxed.

"Give him a kiss, and then let's let Dad rest."

They each kissed their dad's lips, and Cate ushered them out the door.

"Did he really know it was us?" asked Ben.

"He did," said Kayla, her voice clear. "Mom, is that what he's always like?"

"Most of the time. He gets more awake for a while, then he sleeps again. Sometimes he knows me, and sometimes he doesn't."

The children considered that and didn't talk much as they drove home. Cate kept an eye on them in the rearview mirror. To her relief, Ben didn't two-tap, and his body curled comfortably into the seat.

As they neared home, she asked what they thought.

"You're right. He does look like a prizefighter," said Ben.

"He looked dizzy when he walked," said Kayla.

"That was probably the second or third time he's been up after a week in bed. I think his hip hurts."

"Why, Mommy?" asked Ben. "Did he break that too?"

"No, sweetie. Just a bad bruise. It's all black and blue."

"Like his face?" he asked.

"Worse because it's a bigger bruise, but it will get better."

They reached home with barely enough time to use the bathroom before Meg arrived with Evie and David. Meg and her family planned to entertain Kayla and Ben for the day. Cate had signed a permission slip for Ben to try gymnastics; the girls loved it, and the boys wanted to try. After that, they would visit the Minnesota Zoo, a bigger zoo than Como. Ben was eager to see the new black bears on the zoo's Minnesota Trail, and Kayla loved the snow monkeys and the Tropical Reef with colorful fish and big turtles. Because Karen and Dan would spend the day at home in Northfield, Cate could enjoy the rest of the day without pressure. Then Meg and Cate's families and Jeff's parents would reunite at a restaurant for Mexican comfort food.

Cate spent the remainder of the morning puttering around the house, reading the *Star Tribune,* watching blue jays and cardinals at the bird feeder and the squirrels gathered below, eating what the birds knocked from the feeder. A couple of times a day, a squirrel tried climbing the pole to reach the seed but couldn't get past the squirrel baffle. Yet the squirrels kept trying.

At lunchtime, she made herself a ham and cheese sandwich. Then she returned to the hospital, yearning to see significant progress since the morning, knowing she'd be disappointed, brooding about her marriage. She steeled herself for a joust between love and doubt, which would end in neither one unhorsed.

Cate stayed for a few hours. Jeff took another walk with aides, and his eyes opened for a longer time. He stared at the TV, tuned to a children's show, less strident than the news, and seemed to respond more to sound and color than content. Jamar, the nurse Jeff had in the ICU, stopped by to see him and say hello to Cate.

"Hey, buddy. You're on the way," said Jamar with his usual energy and good cheer. "You and your nice family'll do great."

"I keep thinking about what you said when Jeff was still in the ICU about stop-and-go traffic that moves eventually. It's a good description, and it makes me laugh, even on a day that's more stop than go."

"Glad it helped."

"You're a good guy, Jamar. You helped us through a rough time, always patient, good at explaining what seemed so scary and overwhelming." Cate teared. "Calm and competent. You made me feel as safe as any family member could feel in an ICU."

"Well, thanks."

"May I give you a hug?" Jamar opened his arms. "Thanks for all your help."

"You and Jeff take care. And please, keep in touch, Cate."

"I sure will."

Cate left the hospital a couple of hours before dinnertime, needing a break and not sure what to do. Neither home nor work beckoned. A coffee shop felt sterile. She shut her eyes in the parking ramp and let her thoughts wander, a rarity in her goal-directed life.

What came to mind was a trip she took to Florence, Italy, during spring break as a college sophomore. Exhausted, she'd collapsed onto a bench in the New Sacristy in the Basilica of San Lorenzo, not thinking about art or beauty. Yet the harmony of the Medici chapel seeped into her consciousness and washed over her, an extraordinary aesthetic and spiritual experience, which she recalled in striking detail: the wide domed cube of gray sandstone, the four elegant statues, Night and Day, Dawn and Dusk, the exquisite harmony of the Medici chapel designed entirely by Michelangelo. That memory connected Cate to a part of her she rarely accessed.

Feeling dizzy and cold, Cate opened her eyes to cinderblocks and concrete. She started the car and drove, almost without conscious decision, to the Minneapolis Institute of Art and headed for works from the Italian renaissance. She found a seventeenth-century black crayon drawing, the Study of Michelangelo's Night Sculpture, from the Medici tombs, attributed to Cesare Dandini, and planted herself on a flat bench in front of it. It felt good to sit there, thinking about Florence.

* * *

That evening, as Cate and Meg's families and Jeff's parents ate fajitas and enchiladas, the kids talked about bears. "Black bears aren't always black," said Ben.

"Really?" said Karen.

"Sometimes they're gray, light brown, or cinnamon like that stuff we put on toast," said Ben.

"There are white bears, too," said Kayla. "They're called spirit bears."

"But the zoo doesn't have any of those," said Ben.

"They're rare. Most live in Canada," said Evie.

"We saw a picture of one," said David.

Dan asked if they were albinos. Kayla and Evie said they weren't because they were creamy, not white, and their noses, eyes, lips, and paws were dark.

"We did see two black bears and a cinnamon bear," said David. "They were orphans."

"The cinnamon bear's name is Sike," said Ben. Meg had pictures on her iPhone of the children in front of the bears. One showed Kayla and Ben with Sike shaking snow from his cinnamon coat. "Meg emailed it to you, Mommy, so we can give it to Daddy," said Ben.

"I'll print it," said Cate, "and we can add it to Dad's wall."

"Good, Mommy. Daddy will like that."

CHAPTER EIGHTEEN:

Monday, Hospital Day 8

Early Monday morning, Cate reached the neurosurgery floor where Jeff sat in a recliner, his blue bathrobe brighter than his pasty skin. Two feet from the window rose the brick wall of an adjacent building, which made the room dark and unpleasant. Yesterday, Cate had tried to cheer the room, taping to the wall all the pictures that followed Jeff from the ICU.

"Kayla and Ben loved seeing you yesterday," she said. Jeff's chin dropped and rose. "After their visit, they went to the zoo and wanted you to have this picture." She showed him the photo of the kids and Sike and added it to the wall. Jeff smiled, but the room still looked bleak.

Cate missed the hectic energy of the ICU, which made her think of Jamar, who said that it helps to stand back and see the movie and not dwell on every frame. What occurred to her was *Regarding Henry*, a movie about a high-powered attorney shot in the head, his long and imperfect recovery, how he endured, and his family adjusted. It was a different kind of TBI, an open or penetrating injury, not a closed injury, but there were plenty of similarities. Cate looked at Jeff, seated in the recliner, eyes vacant, and tried to feel optimistic.

Jeff's parents arrived at the same time as Jeff's breakfast—oatmeal and an egg, with an aide to feed him. Karen said she'd do the feeding.

Cate observed them, mother and child, and thought of the Gerber baby, its curious eyes, bowed mouth, and lovable smile, a face full of life. Jeff's face held no expression. She had an urge to taste Jeff's food, as she had with Kayla and Ben.

Breakfast concluded, Karen pushed away Jeff's tray, and the daily cavalcade of caregivers began with a physical therapist. Cate remembered Jeff's lumbering strolls yesterday, supported by aides. The therapist guessed that Jeff was probably half awake when that happened. The belt that she used to support him made walking easier, more natural than throwing arms over people's shoulders. She wet a washcloth with cool water, touched the cloth to his wrists and face to chase away grogginess, guided him with the belt out of his room for twenty steps, and returned. As Jeff eased into the recliner, he grimaced and touched his left hip. "I know that hip hurts, but walking won't make it worse," she said. "We're going to do this twice a day, so I'll be back this afternoon."

As Cate surveyed the dingy room, thinking about how to make it brighter, an effervescent nurse appeared, flipped on all the lights, and taped to unoccupied parts of the wall three large, framed pictures of brilliantly colored azaleas, reds and purples and pinks, densely packed on both sides of a hilly path.

"This gloomy room needs some joy, so I always bring a few of my favorite pictures," she said. "Every spring, people come from all over to see these blooms at the National Arboretum, a few blocks from where I grew up in D.C. My name's Azalea, and my mother named me for these flowers. She liked daffodils too, but she didn't want folks to call me Daffy." A laugh as vibrant as the blossoms brightened the dark space. Azalea turned to Jeff. "Now, let's make you comfortable." Jeff seemed to absorb her energy, and his eyes livened as Azalea arranged his blanket and pillows on the chair.

"Did you know we have an arboretum here?" asked Cate.

"Really? We moved to Minneapolis only a month ago. My husband's a safety engineer with 3M."

Cate pointed to the picture of Kayla and Ben in a field of tulips. "That's our arboretum."

"You've made my day, honey. I'm gonna take my family as soon as spring rolls around, if not before." Before Azalea left, Cate showed her the website on her iPhone.

"She's a stitch, isn't she?" Jeff responded with half a smile. Cate turned on the TV news and pulled a chair next to Jeff. They watched, holding hands.

A few minutes later, Dr. Rita Menendez and her bank of swans flew into the room. She told Cate that Jeff had a low-grade fever and a few noises in his chest early that morning that could be pneumonia. Since people with brain injury often have problems swallowing, she had ordered a chest X-ray and a barium swallow to be sure no food reached his lungs. Both were normal. She listened to Jeff's chest, which was clear, noted that his last two temperatures were normal, and announced that Jeff would graduate from critical care free of acute problems. She said goodbye to Cate, wished Jeff well, and left.

The person Cate most wanted to see, had scheduled to see, was Dr. Laura Boulder, the physical medicine doctor who would approve the transfer to Knapp rehabilitation and manage his rehab care, and soon she arrived, a tall brunette with a friendly oval face. Yesterday, she'd examined Jeff and reviewed his chart. "The news is good," she said. "Hopefully, language will improve soon, and he'll be able to recognize people. Then we'll have a lot more to work with, even if he's still confused. He can transfer in a couple of weeks."

"No nursing home?"

"I think he'll be ready." Cate looked at Jeff. Language and recognition seemed a long way off. "I know," said Dr. Boulder, "it's hard to imagine, but he's about to make big strides."

Dr. Boulder had tried a few times to catch Jeff's dad. She handed Cate a business card and invited him to call. With an encouraging smile, she left.

No nursing home. Cate breathed a sigh of relief.

CHAPTER NINETEEN:

Tuesday, Hospital Day 9

Jeff, she learned, had gone for a follow-up MRI. She searched her purse for a picture she'd taken from the photo album the night before—Kayla and Ben at the Minnesota Landscape Arboretum in front of magnificent azalea blooms—and taped it to the wall between Azalea's azaleas and Minnesota tulips. Now the room burst with color despite the lack of sunlight. Olivia poked her head into the room to say the MRI looked good, and the room seemed even brighter.

Jeff arrived, pushed in a wheelchair by a desultory aide, who announced his return by smashing the chair against the doorjamb. Jeff grunted but looked unperturbed as he shifted to the recliner. His eyes found the flowers, all of them, and he seemed to sit taller in the chair.

Cate talked to him about the pictures, telling Azalea's story, reminding him when each of the family pictures was snapped, including the Cape Cod beach picture and the one of Jeff playing Roughhouse. As she talked, Jeff warmed to her voice. The moment she stopped, his eyes grew vacant.

"W … Umm," Jeff muttered and looked at his empty pitcher.

"Are you thirsty?" she asked. "Do you want some water?"

"W …," he said, accompanied by a barely perceptible nod. Cate, afraid to trust her perception, saw Azalea in the doorway.

"Did you hear that?" said Cate.

"He's trying to speak," said Azalea. She fetched more ice water and filled his glass. He drank it down and extended the cup toward the pitcher. She poured another glass, and he drank again. "Any other sounds or words this morning?" asked Azalea. Cate shook her head. "Well, if he's not there, he's close," said Azalea. She spied the azalea picture Cate had added next to hers and chortled. "Can't have too many azaleas. I like your other pictures, too. Nice family."

Cate laughed. "When your mother named you, she got it right."

"Let me try something." Azalea turned to Jeff. "Tell me your name." She waited. "Jeff. Your name is Jeff. Tell me your name."

"J...f..." Cate was not sure if he knew his name or mimicked the sound, but either represented progress. She pulled her chair close to him and touched his arm.

"Jeff, say my name." He pulled back as if to study her. "Cate, I'm Cate." Although his eyes narrowed in concentration, he produced no sound. Cate sat close, her eyes fixed on his, and tried again. Nothing. Azalea reassured her that this was what early improvement looked like. Cate nodded and excused herself, paced the hall, noticed the vending machine, and bought matching diet cream sodas for Jeff and for herself. In the room, Jeff stared at CNN. She opened both cans, put a straw in Jeff's, handed him the can, and took a swig from hers. He put the straw in his mouth and took a sip.

"Thinks," he said.

Cate looked up abruptly and grinned. "You're welcome," she said. But Jeff's head fell to his chest, and he slept.

Cate felt both excitement and an urge to flee the room but stayed and opened her computer. She searched for something easy and engaging and decided to work on an interesting thesis proposal of a new graduate student. Although it was well written, she couldn't concentrate, so she turned to email, which took less effort. She answered several queries from students, attended to a few administrative details, responded to a note from Jennifer about the symposium, and looked through the list of people who'd written and been referred to CaringBridge.

As she worked, an email arrived from Jack Ross. He asked how she was doing and said he was thinking about her, his tone cordial and kind. She read it and thought about how good a run would feel, a release of pent-up tension. She looked quickly at Jeff, whose eyes had opened, and thought about trying again to interact. All she could think of was the joust, the battle between love and doubt.

Jeff reached for his diet cream and sipped. Some remained in Cate's, and she finished it. She decided to fetch two more, but she needed a longer walk. She took her coat and her computer and walked outside, circling the hospital, then sat in the lobby, her computer open but unattended, watching people.

As she returned to Jeff's room, holding two fresh cans of diet cream, she heard whispers and paused outside the doorway, recognizing the voices of Jeff's parents.

"The accident couldn't have happened at a worse time," said Dan.

"I know. If he felt distant, she probably felt the same way. I told him he should talk with her directly," said Karen.

Jeff was feeling distant from me, and he told them? thought Cate. She tried to convince herself that talking with his parents was no big deal, that Jeff and his parents were close. Yet she felt vulnerable and exposed.

She wondered who else Jeff talked to. Maybe Scott? But Scott would probably have told Meg, who would have told her, unless Scott considered the comment confidential. Cate wanted to be fair; after all, she had talked to Meg.

Why hadn't Jeff brought this up to her? Was he also thinking of separation? Nothing about their interactions, their fight, suggested that, but he'd done nothing to bridge the distance. She sensed anew how far apart they'd drifted, how much joint effort it would take for their marriage to repair.

Karen and Dan had remained gracious to her. Their bond felt intimate and real. Perhaps Jeff's discussion with them had described the normal ups and downs of marriage, not a rift.

She took a cleansing breath, forced a smile, and entered the room. To Cate's relief, Jeff's parents greeted her with affection. She opened the can, inserted a straw, handed it to Jeff, and offered the other to Jeff's parents, who declined. She popped open her can and sipped.

* * *

As Karen helped Cate prepare dinner, she offered a heartfelt hug. "You're doing an excellent job managing everything," said Karen.

"You sure are," said Dan.

"I'm glad you're here. I couldn't do it without you," said Cate.

During dinner, Ben mentioned their trip to the zoo. "Hey, I've got an idea," said Kayla. "We could add a spirit bear to the snow family. To help Dad get better."

"Yay, a spirit bear!" said Ben.

"There's fresh snow. Let's add a grandma and grandpa, too," said Kayla.

"That's a lovely idea," said Cate.

When they finished, the spirit bear stood on his hind legs in front of a family of six, its right arm bent, paw against his forehead in sharp salute. More scarves weaved the enlarged family and spirit bear together.

CHAPTER TWENTY:

Friday, Hospital Day 12, December 14

"Out the door. It's late," said Cate. Kayla and Ben paused to look at the spirit bear and snow family and waved to Cate, who watched from the stoop.

Cate had another cup of coffee with Jeff's parents, then worked for an hour in her home office. Whenever Cate had downtime at the hospital, she also worked, which she preferred to reading a book. Work helped maintain equilibrium, protected her family, and no longer felt selfish.

By Friday, Jeff seemed to grasp—some of the time—that he was in a hospital but didn't understand why. When Cate entered the room, he was half-turned toward the TV.

"Hi, Jeff."

"C...Cate." The easy use of her name excited Cate, even if his voice was flat. His left cheek elevated in a partial smile, which meant weakness, drooping, on the right side of his face from damage to the left motor strip in the brain. Cate suppressed a groan; she was learning too much neurology.

Jeff raised his arm and gestured toward his head. "Head … er … I." Olivia had described *expressive dysphasia*—the inability to put thoughts into words, speech that was labored or halting. But he was talking!

"Does your head hurt?" she asked.

He frowned, shifting uneasily in his chair. "Um ... sored."

Olivia had also described *receptive dysphasia*—difficulty understanding spoken language. To Cate's relief, Jeff seemed to understand.

The nurses had coached Cate to converse as naturally as possible and to tell Jeff, over and over, in simple terms, where he was and what had happened. She rested her hand lightly on his arm and repeated words that had become mantric. "Jeff, you're in the hospital. You had a car accident. You have a brain injury."

"Nurse … ah …" His right hand pulled the blanket that lay across his lap into a clenched fist. His eyes widened in frustration.

"I know you're trying to tell me something." His face calmed a bit, and he loosened his grip on the sheet. *I'm reading him correctly,* she thought. "I know it's hard for you to speak. The good part is that you understand."

"Bump … eh …" He exhaled audibly, eyes moist.

Cate put her arms around him. He rested his head on her shoulder.

"Jeff, you had a car accident. You have a head injury."

"Head, bed … say … Shit!"

Cate laughed nervously. Expletives, she'd read, were common with expressive dysphasia.

"Today … uh …?"

"Ten days ago. That's when you had the accident."

"Occ…dint …"

"The doctors say your speech will get better."

"S...say…"

This is starting to feel like a conversation, she thought. "You slept for a few days. Then you started to wake up, but you're still sleepy." She knew he didn't remember any of this.

Jeff moved uncomfortably in the chair and reached for his left hip. Cate thought of his swollen and discolored hip. "Acher," he said.

"You bruised it. It'll hurt for a while."

Jeff reached up and touched the bandage on his head. His brow lowered, narrowing his eyes.

"Sore?"

His brow eased.

"That's where the doctors removed a blood clot."

"Glob. Gob?"

"Inside your skull. They made a hole in your skull to get it out."

"Ooch."

She touched his forehead, avoiding the fracture and bandage. "There are bruises on your brain too."

"Tired," he said. He yawned and looked away.

A real word! She cradled his head against her chest gently because it seemed frail and brittle. "Do you want to watch TV? You were watching when I came in." She lifted his head so she could see his face. His wide-eyed look, the droopy right side of his face, reminded her of an emoji, the confused one with a crooked mouth and vertical ovoid eyes. His chin sank to his chest.

She lingered, watching him sleep.

CHAPTER TWENTY-ONE:

Saturday, Hospital Day13, December 15

Cate led Kayla and Ben down the busy hallway past the open doors of patient rooms. There were several visitors chatting inside them, doors ajar, or talking in the corridor. A woman about Cate's age in a sweater and jeans looked up from a magazine and smiled at the children.

"This visit will be a little longer," said Cate. "Let me know if you have questions."

A half-chewed burger smeared with ketchup, resting on an unattended food cart, caught Ben's attention; he turned away in disgust. Across the hall from the cart, a harsh ray of sun spotlighted the bottom of hospital pajamas, and feet slippered in moccasins that resembled Jeff's.

Ben stiffened. "Is that Daddy?"

"No, sweetie. His room is down the hall," said Cate.

"I don't like that man's feet," said Ben, more anxious than on previous visits. Cate wrapped an arm around his shoulder.

"They're just feet," said Kayla.

"This hospital smells bad," said Ben. "I think it's that hamburger."

"It's not the hamburger," said Kayla. "Someone barfed."

A nurse in blue scrubs overheard her and chuckled. "You're right," she said. "We'll have it cleaned up in a jiffy. By the way, I'm Maude."

"I'm Kayla, and this is my mom and my brother Ben." Cate appreciated her daughter's poise.

"Say, I bet you're Jeff's family." Kayla and Ben beamed. "I'm your dad's nurse. Your dad was wide awake a few minutes ago."

Maude kept them engaged as they continued down the hall. They paused a few steps from an open door, and Maude pointed out Jeff's room. Ben froze. Cate gripped his hand and pulled gently.

"It's okay, Ben. You're going to have a nice visit," said Maude. Ben grabbed the leg of a chair and held tight.

"There's nothing to be afraid of," said Cate. Ben went limp. *Now what?* Cate scooped him into her arms, hugged him, set his feet on the ground, and watched him sink again onto the floor. "Get up, Ben. Hospital floors are dirty."

"You told me hospitals are clean." Ben stared at his mom with suspicion.

"Yes, but floors are dirty everywhere," said Cate.

"Not at home. We play on the floors," said Ben.

Kayla shot Cate a look of disapproval, crouched next to Ben, and extended her hand. "Ben, stand up and we'll walk together." He stood and accepted Kayla's hand but cringed toward her, avoiding the chairs.

"Are hospital chairs dirty, too?" he asked.

"The chairs are clean, Ben," said Maude.

"If they're clean, you can touch them," said Kayla. "See?" She sat in a chair and directed Ben to the chair next to her. Cate took the chair on Ben's other side, and the tension in Ben's face lessened.

"Sweetie, what are you afraid of?" asked Cate.

"That Daddy won't know us," said Ben. "You said he doesn't always know you."

"Sometimes he doesn't, especially if he's tired, but most of the time, he does." Cate tousled his hair, and Ben calmed further.

"That's better. You might have to wake him up, but you're going to have a nice visit," said Maude and left with a reassuring pat on Ben's shoulder.

"Let's go," said Kayla. She took Ben's hand and led him into the room, with Cate following.

Sun filtered through a curtained window and coated Jeff with flaxen light as he slept on the recliner, his bright blue robe open to reveal a clean blue and gray hospital gown. Kayla ran to him and touched his arm. Ben stood behind his mom and peeked around her. "Hi, Dad," said Kayla. Jeff's eyes opened and slowly focused. His cheeks elevated and his lips curled into the most symmetric smile Cate had seen. "Hi, Dad. We came to visit." Kayla waved to Ben, who walked to the other side of the recliner. "See, we're both here."

"Hi, Daddy," said Ben. Tentatively, he touched his dad's face.

"We missed you, Daddy," said Kayla softly.

"Kay-a," he whispered. Cate, who'd held her breath, exhaled. Ben withdrew his hand from his dad's face, but Kayla climbed onto Jeff's lap and pointed to the other side, where there was room for Ben. After a glance at his mom, Ben joined Kayla on his dad's lap. Jeff's arms encircled the children loosely. "Bin-a," he said. Ben burrowed into his dad's embrace, and Cate exhaled again.

"Are you better, Daddy?" asked Ben. Jeff's eyes dulled, his eyelids fell and rose again.

"You're tired, aren't you," said Kayla, with an air of confidence. "I can see your hair is growing," said Kayla, leaning, looking around his head and pointing to shoots of hair on the left.

"You still look funny, Daddy," said Ben.

"C'mon back over here," said Cate, who'd remained on the side of the bed near the door, "where you can't see the shaved part." Ben got down, walked to his mom, and his face brightened. She gave Ben a nudge, and he walked back around the chair and climbed again into his dad's lap. Jeff's eyes had closed.

"I love you, Daddy," said Ben. Jeff did not stir. "Why won't he open his eyes, Mommy?"

"Wake him gently and try again," said Cate. Ben placed a hand on Jeff's arm and shook it until his dad looked at him with a tired smile.

"I love you, Daddy," Ben repeated. Jeff's eyes, at first cloudy, cleared and glowed. Ben grinned from ear to ear and hugged his dad, who put an arm around him and pulled him close. Kayla, imitating Ben, snuggled against him. He turned to look at her.

"I love you too," said Kayla.

"Kay…a...Bin," said Jeff, smiling with his eyes. "Lubbu."

"We all love you, honey." Cate's voice quivered.

"Why are you crying, Mommy?" asked Ben.

"Because Dad's hurt and because I love this visit."

"Sad tears and happy tears," said Kayla softly.

"It's time to go. Dad needs to rest," said Cate. She planted a gentle kiss on Jeff's lips. "I'll bring the kids back soon, honey." The kids kissed their sleepy dad, climbed off his lap, and said goodbye. Ben touched Jeff's arm twice, repeated the two-tap, and stifled a sigh.

"It's okay," said Kayla, wrapping an arm around Ben. Again, they said goodbye. Jeff's eyes flickered open.

"Bye," he said before his eyes slid closed.

With a hand on each shoulder, Cate guided the children to the elevator. Four floors down, they emerged from the elevator and walked into the bracing December chill.

CHAPTER TWENTY-TWO:

Thursday, Hospital Day 18, December 20

Cate awoke before the alarm, disoriented by a nightmare, and peered through the bedroom window at a freezing fog. In the haze of blue and white, a ghostly circle of light pulled a humanoid figure upward, and a shadowy green mesh held it against a translucent floor. She blinked and slapped her cheeks, but the image persisted. Cate walked to the bathroom, splashed cold water on her face, brushed her teeth, and returned to the window, where sunrise had painted residual haze a soft yellow, the color of clarified butter.

She heard the children, called good morning, and descended the stairs to the kitchen. To her delight, Kayla had already made Cream of Wheat, complete with a dash of cinnamon in each bowl. There was even a bowl for Cate. As Ben hurried down the stairs, Cate poured two glasses of milk and started the coffee, then joined the kids at the kitchen island. It could've been a normal morning, one where Jeff left early to implant embryos. They talked about school. As the kids prepared to leave, Ben repacked his backpack twice and said his stomach hurt but recovered quickly. After tomorrow, winter break would begin, and school stress would diminish.

Once the bus rolled from sight, Cate buried herself in a few hours of work. Although winter break had already begun at the university, she continued to find work stabilizing. The morning passed quickly, and the drive to the hospital on a sun-filled morning was pleasant enough.

At one, she met with Jane in Jeff's room for an update. "Good news," said Jane, and smiled at Jeff. "Tomorrow, you transfer to Knapp Rehabilitation Center."

"Now that's progress!" said Cate. Jeff nodded without emotion, and Cate felt a twinge of foreboding, wondering what the next step in recovery might reveal.

Jane had arranged a tour of Knapp that would begin in a few minutes. She suggested that Jeff wear street clothes, which cheered Cate, who helped him into a navy sweatshirt, jeans, and loafers. He was ready when Jane returned, piloting a wheelchair.

"Why does he need that?" said Cate. "He can walk."

"He can, but it's a long trek." Jeff moved to the wheelchair. Jane directed Cate to the handles and said Cate could be the engine. "Once you're in rehab, you'll walk everywhere." Every day had been a succession of parades, thought Cate, as she stepped briskly. Today, she and Jeff would be the marchers.

They marched first to occupational therapy, which looked like an adult children's museum, with a model grocery store and a kitchen with real appliances. They watched a woman, supervised by a therapist, insert plates into dishwasher slots while another therapist guided a man's hand on a knife as he chopped carrots. Jeff's wrist flicked as if he were chopping, and Cate smiled.

Kim, a determined young woman who'd be Jeff's therapist, introduced herself. "Jeff, I hear you're an accomplished cook. I'm going to get you back in the kitchen."

"Cook," said Jeff.

"That's right. We're going to work on all the activities of daily living—what we call ADLs—cooking, dressing, and hygiene. Some of the time we'll practice doing them, some of the time we'll work on planning *how* to do them." She turned to Cate. "We'll break down every task into its parts, perceiving, remembering, thinking. In other words, we'll help Jeff figure out what he knows from his senses, what comes from memory and experience, and how to use that information to get things done."

"I've read about Cognitive OT. Is that what you're describing?" asked Cate.

"Yes. It looks different at different stages of recovery. At this point, I'll see him for a couple sessions each day. We'll do the planning part with paper and pencil."

"Would you like a cookie?" A woman who'd just finished a batch of chocolate chip cookies offered some to Jeff and Cate. Jeff grabbed one from the tray and bit into it.

"Good," he said. "Good cookie."

"Say thank you, honey," said Cate.

"Thank you," said Jeff, with a smile that surprised Cate.

From OT, they walked to SLP, speech and language pathology. The SLP therapist, a lanky man with red hair and a jocular manner, introduced himself as Rudy Herring and said folks called him Red.

"A red herring?" Cate laughed. For one of Jeff's birthdays, she'd given him a set of Learning Company CDs, a linguistics course by Anne Curzan called *The Secret Life of Words*, which they had spent hours discussing. "You remember red herring from our CDs, don't you?" said Cate. Jeff furrowed his brow. "When a guy in England used a red herring to throw hounds off the scent and save a hare?" Cate watched Jeff. He said nothing, but his eyes sparkled as if he understood; he used to love this kind of banter.

"Yup," said Jane. "It's a perfect name for a language guy."

Red would help Jeff choose the right words and form clear sentences.

"That's a lot of info for one day, Jeff. How are you doing?" asked Jane.

"Okay," said Jeff. They accompanied Jeff back to his room, where Cate sat with him for several minutes before kissing him goodbye.

For Cate, the hospital day was not yet over. She had questions for Dr. Boulder, and Jane had suggested she address them without Jeff. When they reached Dr. Boulder's office, she stood to greet Cate. Karen and Dan sat waiting. "Hi, Cate," said Dr. Boulder. "I understand you have questions. How can I help?" Cate took a moment to organize her thoughts.

"Well, I've done a lot of reading. I've seen Jeff's MRIs, but I don't understand what happened to Jeff's brain. I think the term is 'mechanism of injury,' and Jane said you could explain it."

"I can. It will help you understand the severity of Jeff's injury, but it gets pretty graphic." Dr. Boulder hesitated. "Are you sure you want this level of detail?"

"I've thought about it a lot, and I do. I can use a computer or a car without understanding how they work, but Jeff isn't an object to operate or drive. He's my husband. Maybe it sounds nuts to you, but I have to understand what happened to Jeff's brain. I've told everyone, consistently, that information helps me cope."

"Okay," said Dr. Boulder. "Feel free to stop me at any time." Her gaze included Karen, who looked less certain, and Dan.

Dr. Boulder produced a life-size model of a brain and skull that she used to teach students. She removed the top of the skull so that Cate could see how the brain fit inside it, then removed the brain so Cate could see the irregular bony skull floor on which the brain rested. Dr. Boulder pulled from a bookshelf a model car, put the skull in the driver's seat as if it were a person, and wheeled the car across the floor of her office.

"Do you see what's happening? The brain, skull, and person are traveling down the road at the same rate as the car. That's important because what I'm going to show you is based on the physical law of *inertia,* the idea that an object in motion tends to remain in motion. Got that?"

Cate nodded.

Dr. Boulder wheeled the car into the wall. The car stopped, but Dr. Boulder propelled the skull against the windshield of the model car. "That's what happened to Jeff's skull. The car stopped, but inertia carried the skull forward, fractured his skull, and shattered the windshield." Cate and Jeff's parents winced.

"That part is easy to understand. But it's only half of the story." Dr. Boulder repeated the crash with the top of the skull removed so Cate could see the brain. This time, when the skull hit the window and stopped, Dr. Boulder crashed the brain against the inside of the skull.

"See, inertia makes the brain slam against the inside of the skull, just like inertia made the skull hit the windshield."

Again, Cate nodded.

"Have you watched any YouTube videos about brain injury? There are several good ones."

Dan had, but Cate and Karen hadn't. Dr. Boulder pulled one up on her computer. It showed how the brain crashes against the inside of the skull, gets bruised, and then recoils, slamming the brain against the back of the skull, bruising again, causing what neurosurgeons call coup and contrecoup injuries. Cate shivered. Karen gripped Cate's hand, and Dan held Karen's other hand.

"Are you with me so far?"

"I'm with you," said Cate, her voice almost a whisper.

Dr. Boulder removed the brain from the model skull and once again pointed out the irregular floor on which the brain rests. "When the brain shakes violently back and forth, the bottom of the brain, especially frontal and temporal lobes, grate against these bony ridges like clothes on a washboard, causing more bruises. In addition, as the brain shakes, it tears small capillaries inside the brain, causing tiny hemorrhages throughout. The same forces tore the veins on the surface of the brain that caused the subdural hematomas, including the one that required surgery.

"I understand what you've said so far, but what causes those shearing injuries?"

"Good question. That involves another law of physics called *momentum.* Try to imagine a freight train and a car speeding along at sixty miles per hour. Superman tries to stop each one with the same amount of force. Which one would travel farther before it stops?"

"The train?" said Cate.

"That's right. It's heavier and has more momentum. It travels farther."

She showed them the model of the brain and pointed out the gray matter and the white matter. Gray matter contains the cells of the brain and is heavy like the train; white matter has long fibers that connect brain cells to one another and is light like the car. When the brain crashes against the skull, the heavier gray matter travels farther, which shears apart long white-matter fibers, especially where they lie close to gray matter. Dr. Boulder opened her computer to Jeff's MRI and showed Cate the white spots that correspond to these shearing injuries.

"The problem is, even with all our current technology, you can't see the actual cells and connections inside a brain." Dan nodded in agreement. Dr. Boulder paused to give the others time to absorb the information.

"Now, let's talk about healing." Dr. Boulder explained that hemorrhages and bruises in the brain resemble bleeding and bruises anywhere in the body and heal the same way. But in addition, the brain has a special problem. It has to reconnect torn fibers throughout the brain as best it can, despite scarring, and sometimes the brain makes new pathways as well. That can take up to two years. The better these new connections function, the better Jeff's brain will work. "I can't predict the way torn fibers in Jeff's brain will reconnect."

To a limited degree, Dr. Boulder could watch Jeff's brain heal with MRIs. They could measure improvement by serial tests—neuropsychological tests—that evaluate aspects of brain function. But Dr. Boulder couldn't see the cellular damage and couldn't see fibers reconnect.

At the end of the day, what really mattered was what Cate could observe in Jeff's behavior. How well does he remember things, plan, and follow through? What is his personality like? How much warmth and curiosity has he regained?

"So where does that leave us?" asked Cate, gripping Karen and Dan's hands.

"With a lot of uncertainty. It's hard to speculate this early in recovery. Overall, I'd consider this a moderately severe brain injury. That fits more or less with his alertness at the scene and in the emergency room. Two measures that we use to determine severity are how long he was unconscious and when after the accident he starts to remember things. The second is called posttraumatic amnesia. The first is hard to estimate because of the induced coma for agitation, but he starts to remember what happened a few days after the accident."

"Given all that, what's your best estimate?"

"Language is coming back, so that won't be a major problem. Beyond that, whether he'll be able to work, what his personality will be like, I'm not willing to guess. He has a lot of damage, but I've been pleasantly surprised many times." She looked at Dan. "Does that sound about right?"

"I don't have your experience, but it fits what I know." He looked ashen.

"One more thing," said Dr. Boulder, "I'm going to start him on sertraline, an antidepressant. Any questions?"

"Is Jeff depressed?" asked Cate.

"Research shows that medication can minimize depression and anxiety. It's prophylactic."

"I guess that's okay. At least, for the first time, I understand what happened and why Jeff's prognosis is so vague," said Cate. She lowered her head into her hands and cried.

Karen and Dan cried too.

* * *

That night, Kayla, who before Jeff's accident had announced that she was too grownup for bedtime reading, eagerly accepted Grandpa Dan's offer to read them to sleep. Kayla and Ben lay next to each other in Kayla's lower bunk. When the story was complete, Cate rubbed their backs the way she used to do when they were younger. Ben crawled into Kayla's upper bunk, and Cate and the grandparents kissed them goodnight.

Downstairs, Cate poured bourbon over ice for Dan, scotch for Karen and herself, and they talked about the day, staring out the window at the floodlit front yard, where flowing scarves joined the snow family and the spirit bear. Dan finished his bourbon and offered to refresh Karen and Cate's glasses, but they wanted no more alcohol. They sipped what was left and watched the news until they grew tired.

Cate climbed the stairs, flicked on the hall light, opened the door to Kayla's room, and watched the kids sleep. Ben's arm, as usual, hung over the side of the top bunk as if he were reaching for Kayla.

The sound of muffled steps drew Cate's attention. Karen, with Dan beside her, slipped her arm around Cate's waist. They stood for several minutes, watching, before they headed for bed.

CHAPTER TWENTY-THREE:

Friday, Hospital Day 19, December 21

Cate worked through the morning home routines and reached the hospital early, ready for transfer to rehab. Olivia, Dr. Watkins, and the rest of the neurosurgery treatment team gathered in Jeff's room to wish them well. "We can never thank you enough for all you've done," said Cate.

"Bet…r," said Jeff.

"Yes, you certainly are," said Olivia. She and Dr. Watkins shook hands with Jeff and Cate and left. Azalea appeared to help finish packing and gave Jeff and Cate a small picture of her azaleas. "Can't wait for spring to visit your arboretum," she said.

"It's a lovely place with lots to see. Hope it makes you and your husband feel at home in Minnesota."

After several minutes, Jane arrived with a wheelchair to offer Jeff one last ride, and they rolled to Knapp, Cate pushing.

Amy, petite and cheerful, greeted them at the door to Jeff's sunny room and introduced herself as Jeff's primary nurse. His new digs resembled a bedroom, not a hospital room, with a sink, vanity, toilet, and shower. "Jeff, your job here is to become independent, so let's get started." Cate had given him a leather bag for toiletries, and Amy coaxed Jeff to remove the topmost item.

"What is this?"

"Tootbush." He placed it on the vanity next to the sink. He reached into the bag and withdrew a tube, inspected it, picked up the toothbrush, and rubbed the unopened tube against it.

"You've got the idea." Amy opened the tube and helped Jeff squeeze a strip onto the brush's surface.

"What do you call this white ribbon?"

"Tootbush," he said again.

"That was the answer to my last question, not this one." Cate swallowed nervously. Amy, unperturbed, held up the toothbrush and the tube.

"This is a toothbrush. This is toothpaste. You put the toothpaste on the toothbrush to brush your teeth."

"Brush. Paste."

"Say toothbrush and toothpaste."

"Tootbush. Tootpaste."

"Good. You probably brushed your teeth already, but let's do it again." Jeff put the brush in his mouth and licked the paste. Amy moved his hand in a brushing motion against his teeth. Once started, he brushed a few strokes, upper and lower. She encouraged him to finish. Then she handed him a cup of water and asked him to rinse his mouth and spit into the sink.

"Jeff, I'm going to tell you my name again, and I want you to repeat it. My name is Amy."

"Amy."

"In ten minutes, I'm going to see if you remember my name."

They emptied the rest of the toiletries onto the vanity and turned to Jeff's plastic bag full of clothes. Jeff, with urging, hung his shirts and pants in the closet and placed the rest of his clothes in his chest of drawers.

"Okay, what's my name?"

"Amy," said Jeff.

"Very good. You'll need that memory to make use of rehab." Then she asked him to say his own name.

"I'm Jeff."

"Nice. That was a whole sentence. Let's keep going so I can get a baseline." She pointed to Cate. "Who's this?" Cate held her breath; three weeks from the accident, and she couldn't presume a correct answer.

"Cate."

Cate resumed breathing.

"How do you know her?" He wrinkled his forehead.

"My wiff … wife."

"Excellent," said Amy. "Now tell me, where are you? What is this place?"

"Hotel."

Cate tittered because it looked like one.

"Not quite right. This is a place where people get better."

"Hospital."

"Yes. This is a special part of the hospital where people go to restore health. Do you know what it's called?" Jeff looked puzzled. "It's called rehabilitation." He cocked his head, attentive. "Okay, now tell me why you need rehabilitation."

"Head, er, hurt."

"That's right." Amy turned to Cate. "Now I want to see how he reacts to you, how you interact." Cate hesitated, unsure what Amy wanted, but Amy didn't elaborate. Following an impulse, Cate kissed Jeff's forehead, which elicited a smile. She walked around his chair and massaged his neck and shoulders from the back, something they did for each other at times of stress, and felt his elevated shoulders and tight neck muscles soften.

"Ummm," he murmured.

"Nice," said Amy. "You're a good caregiver."

"Thanks, I do my best." But caregiver wasn't a role Cate wanted. She wanted a husband and partner; she wanted the kids to have their old dad back. She moved to face Jeff and cupped his chin. "Honey, I love you. Kayla and Ben love you. We need you. We want you to live a full and happy life."

"That tells me a lot," Amy said. "We'll do everything we can to get him there. What you see is a baseline. Rehab starts today." She pointed to a schedule tucked into a glass holder on Jeff's door. Neither Cate nor Jeff had questions. With an encouraging smile, Amy departed.

Cate and Jeff looked at the schedule together. Jeff shrugged. "I can read it for you, honey. You have OT in half an hour." She suggested a walk in the corridor to acquaint Jeff with his new surroundings. As they ambled down the hall, staff greeted them in a friendly manner. Everyone seemed busy or on their way somewhere, presumably some kind of treatment.

They strolled arm in arm. Cate looked at Jeff and tried to keep her spirits high. She thought about how vibrant Jeff had been twelve years ago on the day they met. He'd marched through the carved oak doors of the Conrad Room at the downtown Hilton wearing a forest green turtleneck in a sea of blazers, talking to another attendee, earnest and confident, handsome and warm. Cate remembered feeling unsettled, trying not to blush. She had thumbed through the biographies each attendee had prepared, trying to identify him. When he described his Peace Corps year in Cuzco, she knew she'd guessed correctly. After the seminar, when he approached her with questions, they conversed easily. She thought about that moment, and the courtship that followed, and pulled Jeff a little closer.

They returned to the room with a few minutes to spare. The TV had a setting for music, and Cate found Django Reinhardt and Stéphane Grappelli playing *Tiger Rag*. They loved gypsy jazz and wished they knew a band in the Twin Cities that performed it.

As they listened, Kim arrived to start the OT evaluation. "I talked with Amy, so I know you can brush your teeth. We can save toileting and showering for when Cate's not here."

"Does that mean we're going to the kitchen?" asked Cate.

"I thought we'd work on dressing, especially since Jeff's still in his pajamas. From now on, you'll get dressed first thing in the morning. What do you want to wear?" He looked toward the closet, then the chest of drawers. "You're looking in the right places." He stood but hesitated. "Which do you want to put on first?" He moved to the chest, opened a drawer, picked out underwear and socks, and looked at Kim, who mimed putting them on. He removed his robe and pajamas, dropped them on the floor, put on the underwear, and sat to pull on socks.

"I'll bet you don't leave your pajamas and robe on the floor at home." He looked at them, puzzled. "Where do they go?" Kim waited. "I'll bet there are hooks in the closet." He found the hooks and draped the garments over them. To his left were chinos on a hanger, but he turned toward Kim. "You can't go anywhere in your underwear, can you?" She smiled. He looked down at his underpants and noticed himself in the mirror. Then he sat in the chair.

"You have to finish getting dressed." Kim took his arm and brought him to the closet; she touched his hand to the chinos, and he pulled them from the hanger. She instructed him on how to thread the belt through the loops; he put on the pants and buckled the belt. "What's next? Don't you need a shirt?" Jeff looked in the closet, but there were none.

"Honey, you just put them in that chest," said Cate. The drawers were full of polo shirts and sweatshirts, nothing with buttons. "He opened a drawer, selected a sweatshirt, and put it on.

"Okay, that's a good start," said Kim. "You know how to dress yourself, but the problem is self-starting and initiative. That's what we'll work on next session." To give Cate and Jeff an idea of what that entailed, she pulled out a worksheet and wrote "Getting Dressed" across the top. She asked Jeff to write below that, "I don't how to start."

"Now that you've seen OT in action, it makes more sense. Sometimes we do things, sometimes we think about how we do them." She gave Jeff an encouraging pat on his shoulder and left.

* * *

In the mid-afternoon, Kayla and Ben arrived from school to find their grandparents packing.

"Don't go," said Ben. "Stay."

"We're going home to free the guest room," said Karen with a smile.

"Who's coming?" asked Kayla.

"Hey, I know, it's Aunt Copper," said Ben.

"Right. And Uncle Paul, too," said Cate. The kids perked up. They loved Cate's younger sister and Jeff's younger brother. "Ben, is it okay if Uncle Paul uses your room?"

"Yes. He can sleep in my bed," said Ben.

"Thanks, sweetie."

"How long will they stay?" asked Kayla.

"The whole weekend," said Cate. They had timed their arrivals to meet at the airport and visit Jeff. "They should be here any minute."

The kids went downstairs and read, watching the windows. When a car door slammed, they sprinted to the front door and opened it.

"They're here!" said Ben.

Copper bear-hugged Kayla and Ben, and Paul lifted them into the air. Ben shouted, and Kayla, abandoning all pretext of dignity, squealed with pleasure.

"You have a red car!" said Ben.

"Isn't it cool? I had to talk Paul into it," said Copper. A red Mustang sat in the driveway.

"It's awesome," said Kayla. The kids grabbed their luggage and carried it upstairs to the guest room and Ben's bedroom while Copper fetched one more bag from the Mustang, a long case with a rounded end. Ben, the first one back to the family room, lit up. "Aunt Copper brought her trombone!"

"Hooray! Play something," said Kayla.

Copper, a ginger-headed version of Cate, six years younger, slightly shorter and more rounded, yet with a toned runner's body, was an accomplished trombonist who played for fun in a jazz band. She assembled the trombone, blasted a riff from *Muskrat Ramble,* and bowed as everyone applauded.

"More," said Ben as Dan arrived with bags of takeout.

"Okay. How about after dinner?" The kids nodded with gusto.

"While Grandpa puts out the food, I'll show the kids what I brought," said Paul. Cate had always liked Paul. He had Jeff's inviting blue eyes and wavy brown hair, but was taller and thinner, built more like Karen, with her quiet charisma.

Paul, who designed wind turbines, had brought Ben a model wind turbine kit and Kayla an award-winning children's book, *Catch the Wind,* that explained how windmills convert wind energy to electricity.

Kayla liked her book and looked wistfully at Ben's model. "That wind turbine would make a good project for my school science fair. After you build the model, can I use it, Ben?" Ben looked doubtful. "I'll let you read my book."

"That way, you'd both learn," said Paul. "If you'd like, I could be your adviser. We could stay in touch with FaceTime or Skype."

"That'd be fun!" said Kayla.

"Okay," said Ben.

"Thanks, little brother." Kayla gave Ben a hug. They sat on the couch next to Paul and read a few pages from *Catch the Wind* until Dan said dinner was ready. Smells of delicious Italian food lured everyone to the kitchen. With food piled high on plates, they headed for the porch, where the topic turned to Jeff.

"He looked good," said Copper. "We used our names like you suggested, but I think he figured out who we were."

"He did, after a while," said Paul.

"Now we're here with you, ready to have fun," said Copper. "We're going to be your mom's maid and butler for the weekend—that is, if Paul figures out how to buttle."

"I can learn."

"I already know how to do maid's work," said Copper. "It's genetic."

"Some feminist," said Cate with a laugh.

"I think men and women are equal," said Kayla.

"Who taught you that?" asked Copper.

"Dad," she responded.

"That's my brother." Paul grinned. "C'mon, Ben, you and Grandpa and Paul can help me rinse the dishes and stuff the dishwasher."

"Aunt Copper, are you gonna give us a concert?" asked Kayla.

"As soon as everyone's ready." She adjusted her shirt from the bottom so that the buttons aligned perfectly and centered her belt buckle. The trombone rested on the family room couch, and she checked to be sure she'd assembled it perfectly. As Cate and Karen tidied the porch and the men stowed the dishes, Copper warmed up.

When her audience gathered, Copper played the *Sesame Street* melody, followed by a jazzy Happy Birthday, and several more tunes, including *Sweet Louisiana,* with muted wah-wahs. Everyone applauded. Cate pulled the creases from her jeans and recentered the buckle.

"Will you play for us?" Copper asked the kids, who'd taken music lessons since they were little. Kayla played piano, and Ben played violin. With all the disruption, they hadn't practiced since their dad's accident.

"I don't feel like it," said Ben.

"I don't either," said Kayla.

"Really? I'd love to hear both of you," said Copper.

"Listening to you is more fun," said Kayla.

"It's okay," said Cate, deciding not to pressure the kids.

"I get it," said Copper. "Sometimes listening is more fun."

"I have an idea," said Cate. She left and reappeared with her violin, sheet music, and a music stand.

Copper looked at the music and grinned. "We haven't played that for a long time," said Copper.

"What is it, Mom?" asked Kayla.

"It's a piece by Elizabeth Raum, *Four Elements for Violin and Trombone*," said Cate.

Copper leaned her sheet music against a lamp, stood back, and adjusted it until it was even. "It has to be just right, or your quirky aunt can't toot," said Copper.

The sisters began to play, hesitantly at first, then with confidence and delight as the violin and trombone toyed with each other. The music moved from earthy jazz to airy hums, to sounds that resembled swirling water and crackling fire. The kids sat on the edge of their seats.

"Bravo!" said Paul.

"Wow, that was great!" said Kayla.

"You play a little better than Mommy, Aunt Copper," said Ben, with a wistful glance at Cate, which drew laughs.

"I play jazz and blues," said Copper. She tucked her shirt in and pulled it straight. "Your mom plays classical music better than I ever could."

Ben looked relieved.

After Copper and Cate stowed their instruments, Kayla invited Copper and Paul to see the photo gallery in the back hall. The kids led the procession through the kitchen door, past the mud room, to walls packed with family pictures from vacations, holidays, and outings. In every picture, Jeff looked vigorous and happy.

Paul stopped at a picture of the children and Jeff talking to a man with a big sword and a swashbuckling hat. "Where did you meet a pirate?" he asked.

"At the Science Museum," said Ben. "It wasn't a real pirate."

"I hope not," said Paul.

"But there was a real pirate ship and real gold treasure," said Ben. Kayla pointed out pictures of the ship, its treasure, and a large bell engraved with *Whydah,* the ship's name.

"I wonder what's at the Science Museum now," said Paul.

"Egyptian mummies," said Ben, looking unhappy. "Daddy was gonna take us."

Paul caught Copper's eye and nodded. "That's where we can go in the red car! Copper and I can take you there."

"Really?" said Ben.

"That'd be fun," said Kayla. "Dad said they had animal mummies, not just human ones."

"And an arch-ologist," said Ben.

"Archaeologist," said Kayla, "videos of real ones at work."

Ben shot his mom a worried glance. "But we have to visit Daddy this weekend."

"You can visit Dad and then go to the museum, maybe on Sunday," said Cate.

"Okay," said Ben.

"Hooray," said Kayla.

CHAPTER TWENTY-FOUR:

Weekend, December 22-23

On Saturday morning, the hospital smelled fresh and clean. No smell of barf. No half-eaten trays of food. A spray of richly colored lilies, some yellow, some deep red, decorated the nursing station, defying winter, and here and there, poinsettias of red and white were visible through open doors of patient rooms.

Cate had filled Jeff's room with several pots of Christmas cactus, their blooms red, some almost purple. Even Jeff glowed with color, his cheeks a healthy pink with only a trace of mottled bruising, his blue eyes shining.

"Good morning, Jeff. I brought Kayla and Ben." Ben yelped and leaped into his dad's lap before Cate could warn him to be careful, but Jeff showed no discomfort. Kayla, to Cate's surprise, clung to her. Cate placed a reassuring hand on her shoulder.

Jeff's eyes focused, and he put an arm around Ben and extended the other arm toward Kayla. "Kayla and Ben," he said softly. Warily, Kayla walked to her dad and hugged him. He put his other arm around her and squeezed. Still tense, she snuggled against him.

No one talked, so Cate jumped into the silence. "See how much better Dad is today?" A stubble of hair had grown enough to obscure the surgical indentation. He'd lost weight, muscularity, and his tan, but was more alert and responsive. Still, no one talked. "Why don't you tell Dad where Aunt Copper and Uncle Paul are taking you tomorrow afternoon?"

"To see the mummies at the Science Museum," said Kayla, "where you were gonna take us."

"Mus…eem," said Jeff.

"They read us your mummy books last night," said Ben. *Bill and Pete Go Down the Nile* was a favorite, and before the accident, in anticipation of the museum visit, Jeff had added *Mummies Made in Egypt* to the bedtime list.

"It was fun, Daddy," said Ben. "But I like it better when *you* read."

"Ben, tell Dad what you'll see at the museum."

"Remember, Daddy, you told us about mummies and the arch-ologist," said Ben.

"Archaeologist," said Kayla, "You keep saying it wrong." She began to speak like a coiled spring unwinding. "Aunt Copper brought her trombone from St. Louis. It has a big slide, but she makes the notes with her mouth like this …" Kayla tightened the sides of her mouth and formed an O, then squeezed her lips together in a horizontal line and sputtered like a trombone mouthpiece. "She changes the pitch with her mouth and with the slide. It's loud and it's funny."

"It sounds like this," Ben interrupted, making his voice as low as an eight-year-old could go, and rumbled a toot.

Kayla kept talking. "She played a duet with Mom. Uncle Paul is nice, but he's not as funny as Aunt Copper. He sounds like you, and he looks like Grandma Karen …" She stifled tears and paused. "Oh, Dad, I wish *you* could take us to the museum."

Cate watched, almost relieved to see her daughter show her distress, and placed a reassuring hand on Kayla's shoulder.

"Lubbu," said Jeff.

Kayla held her dad's hand and looked at him, her cheeks damp. "I'm glad you're coming home on Christmas, even if it's just for a visit. I want you to get well and come home for good."

"Yes, Daddy," said Ben.

Jeff looked confused.

"Christmas is in three days, and you're coming home for a visit," said Cate.

"Home?" he said. Visit?"

"That's right, Daddy." Ben burrowed deeper into his father's lap, and Kayla stepped closer.

"Jeff, we're thrilled that you'll be home on Christmas Day," said Cate. She watched Jeff hold the kids close. After a little time had passed, she said, "Honey, we don't want to wear you out, so we're going to say goodbye, but we'll be back tomorrow. Copper and Paul will be here soon."

"Yesterday," said Jeff.

"That's right, honey. You saw them yesterday. You'll see them today and tomorrow; then they're going home to their own families for Christmas, and you'll be with us."

"Walk," said Jeff as the kids reached for their coats.

"Do you mean we're going to walk, or you want to walk?" asked Cate.

"We."

"Okay, before we leave, let's go for a walk," said Cate. Kayla and Ben, one on each side of their dad, guided him into the hall, and Cate followed. They walked to the end of the long corridor and back, settled Jeff in his room, exchanged hugs, and Cate and the kids left.

* * *

Shortly after the three of them reached home, Meg and Scott arrived with their children. Meg had suggested a run to burn off steam, and Scott offered to take the kids to the mall.

"You look like a pair of bumblebees," he said. Cate and Meg wore identical yellow and black running suits bought for the Dallas Marathon, a trip abandoned after Jeff's accident. If Cate could find time to train, they hoped to wear the suits for Grandma's Marathon in Duluth in June.

"Have a good run but be careful; it's icy," said Scott.

"The paths should be clear," said Meg.

Cate and Meg jogged out of the cul-de-sac, along residential streets and the highway frontage road to the plowed trail behind the nearby shopping village. It'd been over three weeks since Cate's last run, and her legs felt rubbery but limbered quickly, and her breath came more easily than she expected. Once they reached the plowed path and accelerated, she felt the familiar runner's elation.

They'd run for almost forty minutes and were heading home when Cate caught her toe on an elevated root and fell hard, twisting her right knee and landing on her left hand and forearm. "Shit, shit, shit," Cate muttered as she pushed herself up from the ground.

"Wow. That looked bad," said Meg. "Are you okay?"

After taking inventory—she could move everything, but her knee was slightly sore, and her left wrist hurt—Cate looked up and gazed through a thicket of leafless branches at white clouds and an azure sky. "I was afraid of a face plant as I went down, but I'll be all right. You should come down here; it's beautiful, like an abstract painting."

Meg snorted. "Really?"

Cate did a careful sit-up, relying on her abs, then leaned forward with legs crossed beneath her and stood without using her arms, and her knee complained only a little. She used her mittened hands to swat snowy dirt from her butt, winced, and grabbed her left wrist. Meg stepped in and wiped the dirt from her arms, legs, and back. Cate's knee started to hurt more, enough to cause a limp as she ambled toward a stump, sat, removed her mittens, and examined her left wrist. It looked okay but was starting to throb, and movement caused a knifelike pain.

Meg suggested urgent care. "With that knee, can you walk home?"

Cate stood and shifted weight from one leg to the other; the knee felt better, and the limp diminished after several steps. "I don't think the knee's a problem." She sat again and tried to move her left wrist. It hurt. She put on her left mitten, supporting the injured wrist with her leg, using her right hand, but could not use her left hand for the other mitten.

"Let me do it." Meg slid the mitten onto her hand. Cate moved her left hand, flinched, and started to sniffle.

"It feels like the last straw when my body fails me." She glared at her injured wrist.

"Nothing like an injury to make you vulnerable."

Cate's face reddened with anger. "It's not just that. You know, all my life, I made careful choices. When you do that, life is supposed to work. I took a super job in the same city as my best friend, married a great guy, picked a nice neighborhood with the best schools for my kids." She slammed her right fist into her thigh. "Fuck. It isn't fair!" She let herself cry until she felt better. With a head shake, she wiped her eyes and managed a wry smile. "Listen to me, complaining like an adolescent, feeling sorry for myself."

"Maybe that's okay."

"All it does is make me feel guilty. Dear God, Jeff's the one who deserves a good life. And the kids, they shouldn't have to deal with this." Cate sat, holding her wrist. The pain felt almost welcome. Without thinking, Cate reached for a rock near her left foot, but her wrist protested.

"Here." Meg placed the rock near Cate's toe. Using her good knee, Cate managed a short punt into the woods. "Nice kick."

Cate laughed, a giggle, then a chortle. "That *did* feel good." She made room on the stump for Meg, and they sat for several minutes, listening to the quiet of the woods.

In the distance, a series of raucous, piping chirps erupted. Very close to them, a rhythm of similar chirps responded. They looked upward and saw a pileated woodpecker, a magnificent, red-crested bird well over a foot in length, just a few yards above them. Cate had never seen one so close. As they watched, it drummed, its head pounding like a pneumatic drill, haunting and beautiful. It repeated the drumming and flew away, leaving the woods silent once again, and Cate pensive.

They sat until Meg spoke. "Ready to walk home?"

As they headed back, Cate used her iPhone to tell the kids that she hurt her wrist, that Meg would drive her to urgent care. She wanted Kayla and Ben to hear her voice, firm and confident, and know she was okay.

* * *

Cate entered the kitchen wearing a sling on her left arm. Ben, instantly alert, bolted to her side. "Are you hurt, Mommy?" His voice shook. "Don't be hurt, Mommy."

"Did you break your arm?" asked Kayla.

"A sprain and maybe a hairline fracture, not enough for a cast."

"Let me look," said Dan. He stepped around the children and examined her arm. "They should have told you to use it, just avoid anything that hurts."

"That's exactly what they said. And come back if the pain gets worse," said Cate.

"Don't go to the hospital, Mommy," said Ben. He ran to Cate and hugged her.

"Urgent care isn't the hospital, sweetie," said Cate. "You've been there a million times for sore throats and earaches. Kayla too."

"Mom will be fine," said Dan. "Don't worry."

"They can't help but worry," said Karen. She wrapped the children in her arms, and the room grew still. Meg and her family took the opportunity to say goodbye and leave.

Dinner was still a few hours away, and Ben wanted to watch TV. "I have a better idea," said Paul. "This is a good time to talk about wind energy." Both kids, excited, followed him into the family room.

With Kayla and Ben on either side of him, Paul pulled a toy propeller from a briefcase. He asked each of them to blow on the propeller and describe what they saw. Cate smiled, glad to see the kids learning. It reminded her of Jeff describing cow embryos.

"The propellers catch the wind and turn," said Ben.

Kayla had learned in school that a fan uses electricity to turn the blades to make a breeze. A wind turbine operates like a backward fan, turning wind energy into electricity. Kayla wanted her science project to explain how a backward fan works, how wind energy helps the environment; she wanted to understand it well enough to answer questions at the science fair. Watching from the doorway, Cate beamed. Making complex ideas understandable was a skill she and Jeff valued.

As they worked, Paul asked her to list the issues that her project should address. She wanted to show how a windmill converts wind energy into mechanical energy, which turns a generator to make electrical energy. She wanted to explain where the electricity goes once it's made, how electricity is stored, why windmills had to be so tall, and how wind energy compares to fossil fuels and atomic energy. "Those are dynamite questions," said Paul.

"Will you help me build the windmill?" asked Ben.

"Sure. We can work on that tomorrow.

As they put the science project aside, a trombone tooted. "Okay, guys, windmill time is over. It's trombone time."

"Same thing," said Paul.

"What do you mean?" asked Kayla.

"A trombone turns wind energy into sound waves," said Paul. "When you play, you're modifying the waves."

"Uh-oh," said Karen, grinning.

He's just like Jeff, thought Cate.

"Enough learning," said Copper. "It's just music." She played several tuneful riffs. Then the kids laughed as she showed them the mute that made the crying wah-wah sound and other mutes that made hollow or rich or buzzy sounds. Copper wanted the kids to have fun.

After dinner, Grandma and Grandpa kissed everyone goodbye and left for home. Paul fixed the squeaky door to Ben's room, swept the garage, stacked the cord of firewood he'd ordered early that morning, and filled the large wicker basket next to the fireplace with wood and the brass bucket with fatwood kindling.

* * *

While Paul worked and the kids played, Cate had a quiet moment with her sister, who sat with a newspaper carefully centered on her lap.

"What do you make of Ben's two-taps?"

"He's an anxious kid." Copper pinched her earlobes between her thumbs and fingers and rubbed them three times.

"He's a lot like you, and they're starting to get in his way. On school mornings, he gets sick sometimes, and nothing is ever good enough."

"You're worried he has obsessive-compulsive disorder, like me?" Copper had to have her blouse tucked in, buttons straight, belt buckle centered on her jeans, and her hair combed precisely. As a teen, these symptoms had derailed her. Now she managed her OCD with mindful awareness, skills learned in psychotherapy, and medication. She laughed at herself and punctuated her compulsions with humor.

"Yes."

"I've been observing him, and he does have my quirks," said Copper. "It's not surprising that they showed up at a stressful time. Cate, he'll learn to live with his habits and perfectionism if he gets the right help. What helped me was therapy and Prozac."

"They wouldn't give Prozac to Ben. He's only eight."

"I'm a pediatric nurse, and I see lots of young kids on Prozac. It's the medication of choice for OCD."

Cate shook her head, unconvinced. "Isn't that an antidepressant, like the sertraline that Jeff takes?'

"It's the same kind of antidepressant, but Prozac is better studied in kids. A good child psychiatrist would discuss medication pros and cons with you."

"Will you talk to Ben? He loves you." If he did have OCD, Cate couldn't ask for a more reassuring role model than Copper. Her sister had a lovely family and a successful career as a head nurse and nursing school instructor who'd won several teaching awards.

"I already did, yesterday." She'd taken Ben aside, talked about her foibles, how she didn't let them interfere with her life, and what she'd done to get help. "I think he was relieved," said Copper.

"Did you call it OCD?"

"Yup. I named it. I told him a name makes it less scary."

* * *

The next morning, Cate awoke early, disturbed by the idea of medication. *Would they really put an eight-year-old on Prozac?* she wondered. She opened her computer, searched the internet, found it replete with warnings about suicidal thoughts in kids on antidepressants, and resisted the urge to slam the computer shut. She searched further and found opinions by psychiatrists and other experts that antidepressant benefits outweighed risks and helped kids with OCD, depression, or both. The FDA had issued a warning about increased suicidal thinking for people under twenty-five.

At the first opportunity, Cate cornered Copper. “Prozac sounds dangerous. It scares the hell out of me.”

“A good child psychiatrist would talk to you about your concerns. They’d help you weigh the pros and cons.

“It makes kids suicidal.”

“Actually, there’s no evidence of that. Suicidal thinking is a symptom of depression. No one has looked at kids before and after medication to see if Prozac really brings it on. The FDA is being cautious, but they’ve not found any cases of actual suicide.”

“Do you think Ben needs medication?”

“Look at him. He’s such a good kid, with so much potential, but he’s in real pain. He needs all the help he can get.”

Cate shook her head.

“Look, I didn’t get help until my twenties, and I would’ve had a far better childhood with treatment. When I finally took Prozac, it controlled the symptoms. I needed medication to make use of therapy.”

“There are side effects.”

“I know. It can make kids sleepy or irritable, maybe restless. Some kids have trouble sleeping. I didn’t have any side effects, but everyone’s different. If Prozac doesn’t work or causes problems, there are other meds.”

“I still don’t like the idea.”

“You could try without it, see what therapy does by itself. But those habits that are so distressing to him and to you—the two-tapping, checking and rechecking everything, throwing up in the morning, all his perfectionism—they’re exactly the symptoms that Prozac helps.”

Cate sighed.

“It’s winter break. You have time to think about it.”

“I want to see how he does in school after the holidays.”

"That's a good idea, but it won't hurt to make the appointments. When I talked with Ben, he was relieved that help was available."

"That's good to know, but all I can say is, I'll think about it."

* * *

On Sunday afternoon, the kids burst into the kitchen. "Mommy, we saw a mummy chicken!" said Ben, his voice excited. "And livers in canopy jars."

"Canopic jars," corrected Kayla, "separate jars for every organ for the people mummies. Except the heart. They keep that inside the body."

"They do?" asked Cate.

"They thought someone might weigh the heart in the afterlife to see if the mummy had a good life. Bigger hearts are better," said Kayla.

"Then we went to the cafeteria, and a big dinosaur watched us eat lunch," said Ben.

"Diplodocus. It ate plants," said Kayla.

"Hope you didn't eat a mummified chicken," said Cate.

"Yuck," said Ben, and Kayla laughed.

They talked some more about the mummies and how much fun they had. The kids were sad that Copper and Paul had to leave, but tomorrow was Christmas eve; late flights would allow them to leave that evening. The kids helped Copper and Paul pack. Copper had brought a large suitcase because all her mutes did not fit in her trombone case.

After they carried the luggage to the red Mustang, everyone gathered around the snow family and the spirit bear, which the kids had kept in good shape, padding and repairing it with Grandma Karen's help. Jeff's parents, who would once again inhabit the guest room, had joined them for dinner.

They all stopped at the hospital so Paul and Copper could see Jeff once more before they left. For the next hour, they talked about Christmases, past and present, as Cate held Jeff's hand. Jeff seemed to grasp, at some level, that the conversation was about family.

CHAPTER TWENTY-FIVE:

Tuesday, Christmas day

Jeff rose from the wheelchair mandated by hospital rules, locked and held in place by Amy at the hospital door, and walked with Cate and the children to Cate's car parked in the pickup loop. He fumbled at the car door, unsure what to do. Cate put his hand on the handle and showed him how to pull it open, guided him into the passenger seat, and secured his seatbelt as the children climbed into the backseat. "Everyone set?" she said from the driver's seat. Jeff seemed to nod, which evoked a hopeful smile from Cate. Kayla, who sat directly behind her dad, patted his shoulder.

"You're coming home, Daddy," said Ben.

"Okay, everyone, wave to Amy and we're off." As she pulled away, glancing in the rearview mirror, Cate saw Ben two-tapping. "Hey buddy, talk to Dad."

"Hi, Daddy," Ben said, his voice barely audible.

"Tell him about the snow family," said Kayla.

"You have a picture of it, Daddy, but the real snow family is in our front yard, waiting for you."

"Grandma helped us keep the snow family patched up and looking good," said Kayla.

Jeff turned to look at him and Kayla. "Family," he said, with some emotion.

"I'm glad you'll be home for Christmas, Daddy. Grandpa and I got a fire ready with logs and kindling, and Grandpa's gonna light it before you get home."

As Cate eased into the garage, they could smell the fire. Jeff didn't seem to notice as his eyes explored the garage, gazing across the empty parking space at the new cord of firewood that Paul had stacked. He exited the car without help and paused in front of Ben's Quarter Midget racer.

"That's the car you bought me," said Ben.

Jeff's lips twitched but formed no words, and his gaze ping-ponged between Ben and Ben's car as if trying to find purchase.

"Jeff, you're home. This is our garage," said Cate. Daylight streamed through the open garage door and a window. In a voice steadier than she felt, Cate pointed out the things Jeff had noticed—Ben's racer, the firewood stacked along the wall—hoping that repetition would cement him to his surroundings. She pointed to her car parked in its usual spot and to the door to the mudroom. Jeff surveyed the space and seemed to orient himself.

"This is our key," said Kayla. "Watch me unlock the door." She darted up the two concrete steps, flung open the door, and pointed. "See, Dad, you're home. Come in."

Jeff followed Kayla up the steps. She showed him the coat hook and helped him hang up his down jacket. Jeff watched as everyone hung up their coats. Then he walked around the mudroom that doubled as a laundry room and touched the washer and dryer; he seemed to notice the pantry, folding doors ajar, and touched the cans and boxes of food, the paper goods, the spare coffee pot.

Kayla ushered him into the kitchen. He walked to the kitchen island and rested a hand on the granite counter. He seemed to notice the stove directly in front of him, and his eyes took in the cabinets, the sink, the refrigerator, and the four-season porch. He took a few steps onto the peninsular porch and peered through the tall windows as if captivated by the glistening snow and the rolling hills beyond.

"That's the golf course. Isn't it pretty?" asked Kayla. "You and Mom don't play because you think golf is a waste of time."

Jeff's head bobbed as if he agreed. He moved closer to the windows that overlooked the patio and peered through the neighbor's split rail fence. Then he turned and seemed to study the porch itself. Sunlight threw the black and white patterns into sharp relief and highlighted the colorful accent pillows. He sat, and his elevated shoulders seemed to ease. Cate and the kids watched, letting him acclimate.

Jeff looked again at the children, and his face crinkled into a smile. "Home," he whispered.

"Come see more of it," said Kayla. She took his arm and guided him through the kitchen to the family room. Ben followed. At first, the flickering fire caught Jeff's eye. Then he noticed his mom and dad, who stood to hug him. He clung to them, like a small child gaining strength from parents, his face growing calm.

Kayla waited. Then she guided him to the window. There in the front yard stood the snow family.

"Picture," said Jeff.

"Yes, but the snow family is real," said Ben.

They donned coats and walked outside. Kayla took her dad's hand and touched it to each of the figures and to the spirit bear.

"This is you, Daddy," said Ben. He pointed to his dad's red scarf and floppy fedora. Jeff lifted the fedora from the snow figure and put it on his head. "You can have it now, Daddy, but when you go back to the hospital, the snow daddy needs it back." Jeff wore it when they returned to the family room. He took a chair near the window and looked out at the snow family.

Kayla disappeared into the living room and returned with a clay bear she'd sculpted with Karen's help and painted creamy white with darker eyes, nose, lips, and paws. "I made this spirit bear for you," she said.

Jeff held it in his hands. Kayla pointed to the tree, and Jeff placed the bear next to the other presents.

"Do you know what spirit bears do, Daddy?" said Ben. Jeff's eyebrows raised. "They help you get better. We learned that at the zoo."

"That's right, they give you strength and healing," said Kayla.

A log shifted in the fireplace, and a hint of smoke escaped as the flames leaped. Jeff responded to the sound and watched the fire. Cate yearned for him to sniff, to lecture about toxic particles, to adjust the glass doors. Instead, he stared.

Cate also stared. She gazed at the spirit bear that Kayla had made, lying beneath the tree, and hoped.

* * *

Cate sat beside Jeff and stroked his thigh, waiting for dinner. She made small talk, making sure to include Ben, while Kayla and Grandpa helped Grandma in the kitchen. When the fire ebbed, Ben helped his dad add a log. At first, Ben had to guide his dad through each step—stand, walk to the fireplace, open the glass doors, open the metal screen, pick up the wood, add it to the fire, close the doors—but eventually, Jeff performed the steps with less instruction and smiled when the flames jumped and the wood crackled.

By midafternoon, mouthwatering smells emanated from the kitchen—turkey and stuffing, roasted chestnuts, garlicky brussels sprouts, onions, cloves, and cinnamon—and blended with the pine fragrance of the decorated tree and the lingering hint of fireplace smoke.

"Do you smell dinner?" asked Kayla from the kitchen doorway. Jeff didn't seem to understand, which surprised Cate because Jeff loved the smells of Christmas. Usually, he helped make them. Then she gulped as it hit her.

Jeff couldn't smell.

Cate had read that TBI could damage the olfactory system and cause loss of smell but hadn't related that to Jeff. It was a huge loss. Jeff loved the aromas of cooking, the bouquet of a good cabernet, the fragrance of summer woods after a rainfall. The doctors had said that Jeff would gradually reconstruct his world from fragments of memory and sensation; Jeff would have to do that without one of his five senses. Cate thought about how much smell contributed to taste. Could Jeff even enjoy Christmas dinner?

Kayla took a deep sniff through her nose and asked again, "Don't you smell it, Dad?" Cate watched, hoping he might agree, but he didn't, and her heart hollowed.

"My sweet," she said gently to Kayla, "I think Dad lost his sense of smell in the accident. Sometimes that can happen from a brain injury."

"Will it come back?" asked Kayla.

"I don't think so."

"What's it like when you can't smell?" asked Ben.

"Pinch your nose, keep your mouth closed, and try to sniff. Kayla and Ben did that.

"It's weird," said Ben.

"I remember what it smelled like before," said Kayla. "Don't worry, Dad. You just have to remember. It smells like Christmas."

Kayla took her dad's arm, gestured for Ben to take the other, and they escorted him into the kitchen where Karen and Dan had laid out the food. Kayla helped her dad fill his plate and, once he was seated at the table, cut his turkey and vegetables into manageable pieces. Ben squeezed into the empty chair between his father and grandfather.

Cate watched them, three generations of men, and smiled despite the heaviness in her chest. Jeff looked good in the Minnesota Twins cap that Cate had selected; it covered the shorn part of his head. In December, if Jeff were choosing, he would have donned his Vikings cap, but Cate couldn't stand the thought of battered football heads.

Jeff seemed to favor crunchy root vegetables; perhaps it was the texture. He ate as if he were hungry, but without pleasure. Kayla and Karen kept the conversation going, involving Jeff, including Ben. Cate sat quietly at the table, picking at her food.

"Aren't you hungry?" asked Karen.

"I'm just thinking."

"Mom, everything tastes delicious," said Kayla.

"Yes, Grandma did herself proud," said Cate, glancing at Jeff. "Thanks, Karen." She dug into her food, thinking about the allure of taste and smell, enjoying them, and feeling sad.

"Stay home with us, Daddy. Don't go back to the hospital," said Ben.

"Dad has to go back to the hospital so he can get better," said Kayla. "Then he'll come home for good."

Cate had planned to take Jeff around the house—the children's bedroom, their bedroom—but decided it would be too much. Instead, after dinner, all six of them played a couple of games of Clue. Kayla and Ben took turns partnering with Dad, helping him.

At half past eight, Cate helped Jeff into his coat for the drive to the hospital with Kayla and Ben. Dan joined them so he could wait with the car near the hospital door while Cate and the kids trooped to the rehab unit, signed Jeff in, and settled him into the room.

"It was a good Christmas, having you at home, honey," said Cate as she drove.

"Really nice," said Kayla.

"Wish you didn't have to go back to the hospital on Christmas," said Ben.

"Christmas," said Jeff with a smile. "Christmas."

CHAPTER TWENTY-SIX:

The Friday after Christmas, Hospital Day 26, December 28

After a quick trip to the hospital with Kayla and Ben, Cate picked up Meg and her kids, and headed to Nickelodeon Universe, a huge amusement park in the center of the Mall of America. The moms bought passes for the kids, a few tickets for themselves and started at the carousel, a central place to meet if they got lost.

"Let's take the first ride together," said Cate, heading to the entry gate.

"The merry-go-round's boring," said Ben.

"I see a giraffe," said David. Ben brightened. As soon as the gate opened, he raced to the giraffe and climbed on. David rode the zebra, the girls chose a rabbit and a cat, and the moms rode lacquered horses. The bright lights, garish colors, and carousel music pleased almost everyone, but Ben looked disappointed.

"My giraffe didn't go up and down," he said.

"He's too tall," said Kayla. "That camel looks like more fun. You can sit between the humps." Ben looked doubtful but circled back to the entry.

"This time, I want the zebra," said Evie.

"The rooster," said David. Kayla surveyed the animals and chose the lion. The moms stood outside the gate, watching.

"Coney Island. Palisades Park. Swooping roller coasters. I grew up at places like this," said Meg.

"The merry-go-round's thrilling enough for me."

"You like real animals, not lacquered ones," said Meg, grinning.

"To visit, not to ride. I used to spend all day at the St. Louis Zoo, then go home and watch Marlin Perkins and *Wild Kingdom*."

"I loved that show too. It ended when I was twelve, and I missed it."

Cate laughed. "The zoo kept growing, and I kept going."

The carousel stopped, and the kids approached. "Was the camel more fun?" asked Cate.

"A little," said Ben. The kids wanted action. Cate and Meg led them to the tamest of the three roller coasters, which they rode together. Then the girls, tall enough to ride without restrictions, wanted to peel off on their own.

"Okay, if you promise to stick together and not talk to strangers," said Cate.

"Mom, I know that," said Kayla.

"Meet us at the big roller coaster at half past eleven," said Meg. "We can ride that together before lunch."

"The log chute. I want to ride the log chute," said David.

"So do I," said Ben, but his voice lacked enthusiasm.

"Okay, it's the roller coaster and log chute at eleven thirty," said Meg. After that, Scott planned to join them for lunch.

"It's almost time for SpongeBob and Squidward," said Meg, but the moms and boys never got there because they passed the large bumper cars. Ben perked up, especially when he stood in front of the ruler at the entrance; at fifty inches, he could ride alone. He drove cautiously at first, counterclockwise with the flow, avoiding collisions. On his second ride, he began smacking into the rears and sides of other cars and bolted back to the entry gate when the ride ended. David followed.

"Boys and cars," said Meg with a grin. But Ben, eyes glaring, lips narrowed, aimed for the front of another car, and the loudspeaker blared, "No head-on collisions." Ben continued to crash as much as possible. When the ride was complete, he left his car and stalked off, neck red and hands fisted. Cate kept him in sight. She gave him a few minutes of space, then approached and put a hand on his shoulder. He looked at her and said nothing. Then his eyes reddened, and he leaned against her. Gently, Cate patted his shoulder, and he turned, squeezing her and sobbing.

"It's all right, honey," she said, enfolding him in protective arms.

After that, they walked for a while, sampling arcades and shops, playing miniature golf, and riding the Ferris wheel. David seemed to sense Ben's need for solitude, but gradually they began to play and banter. They headed for rides that climbed and plummeted, looped and spiraled, and the boys yelped with pleasure as the moms who sat beside them—most of the rides required chaperones—squealed. When the boys paused for snacks, the moms thought about Pepto-Bismol.

At the designated time, they met at the giant roller coaster and found the girls excited, talking about the platform that had lifted them sixty feet in the air and catapulted them toward the ground. "Hey, we missed that one," said David.

"You're not big enough," said Evie. It turned out that the boys were also too short for the largest of the three roller coasters, even with chaperones, so they wanted an extra ride on the log chute.

Everyone needed a respite before eating. Because Scott was running late, they headed to The LEGO Store. The boys loved LEGO bricks. Earlier that year, the company had introduced LEGO Friends aimed at girls, so Meg thought that Kayla and Evie might like them too. It turned out that the new LEGO Friends were designed for younger girls, with gender stereotypes that the moms disliked, so Kayla and Evie found a bench just outside the store and opened their cellphones.

Aware of Ben's show of emotion, Cate studied Kayla, who seemed removed. Cate joined her. "How are you doing, sweetie?"

"Sometimes, even when I'm having fun, I feel really sad. Mom. What will happen if Dad doesn't get better?"

"We'll make the best of it, sweetie, and we'll be fine."

Kayla nodded, but her mood remained solemn.

Scott arrived and helped the boys build a huge hedgehog. He bought Ben a Ninjago Jungle Raider and David a Ninjago Blaster Bike. The girls didn't want any LEGO toys.

Then they headed to Johnny Rockets for lunch.

CHAPTER TWENTY-SEVEN:

The following Monday, December 31, Hospital Day 36

During winter break, Cate had pushed everything aside except family. With the symposium in two weeks and her mind buzzing throughout the night, she kept a pad on her bedside table to jot down insomniac thoughts.

Now life would resume in earnest. Because Karen had to return to work, she and Dan had abandoned the guestroom. Fortunately, the remainder of Mandy's senior year involved independent study and flexible hours, so she could increase nanny time, help in the mornings, get the kids to and from activities, and make sure they didn't spend endless hours at home alone. Mandy might have to work on her computer while the kids read or did homework, but Cate knew she'd provide a good balance of fun and work.

There was one element of Mandy's presence that troubled Cate. Mandy, at the recommendation of Cate and Rosie, her sister, had asked Jack Ross to sponsor her senior project, which involved frequent contact with Jack. It felt like Mandy's work brought Jack into Cate's house. It bothered Cate enough to discuss it with Meg.

"You work with Jack. What's the difference?" asked Meg.

"It's hard enough to keep him out of my head."

"You're kidding, right? Mandy isn't the issue. You have to figure out what you want from Jack. And what you don't."

On the first post-vacation morning, Cate set her alarm for five and spent the early hours organizing and prioritizing, a strategy she often used when pressure built. Besides work, including the symposium, and her determination to make home as normal as possible, she had to check in with Bonnie, the school counselor, attend Jeff's rehabilitation treatments to get a better sense of his difficulties and progress, and begin to plan for Jeff's discharge, which would entail supervision 24/7 and transportation to and from outpatient rehab.

It was a relief to hear Mandy puttering in the kitchen, getting the kids ready for school as Cate got dressed before joining everyone at breakfast. Kayla, even Ben, seemed happy, eager to return to school. Once they were gone, she gave Mandy a thank-you hug and scurried out the door.

As Cate drove to HCMC on a cloud-filled morning, a fresh dusting of snow contrasted with gray sky. She inserted a CD of Holst's *The Planets,* a gift from Jeff on their first anniversary, the 1986 Charles Dutoit version that he considered the best. After the first few bars of *Mars, Bringer of War,* she skipped to *Venus, Bringer of Peace,* with its lovely solo horn and woodwinds. The snippet of *Mars,* its percussive frenzy, and enchanting *Venus* opened the door to a flood of marital memories—the fire of attraction, the quietude of comfort and trust, disappointments and frustrations, the passion that lingered beneath the surface and emerged with regularity—all of which deepened their relationship and made it real.

As she approached downtown Minneapolis, Cate could see a tiny corner of the Sculpture Garden of the Walker Art Center. She and Jeff had married there more than eleven years ago on a beautiful Sunday in May, when life seemed magical and full of hope. Jeff was wickedly handsome in a black tux. Cate was in a beaded white gown that hugged her toned figure, the same gown that her mother had worn on her wedding day. Meg was also in white beside Cate, two brides, maids of honor to each other, a double wedding. Scott matched Jeff, two grooms, two best men. The nuptials took place beside the iconic sculpture that symbolized Minneapolis, Spoon Bridge and Cherry—the spoon by Claes Oldenburg, the cherry by his wife, Coosje van Bruggen, spouses and collaborators. The brides and mothers wore dresses laced with red that matched the cherry red of the sculpture. Grooms and fathers wore cherry red ties and pocket squares.

Cate thought about meeting Jeff at the first seminar that she taught in Minnesota—how Jeff's thoughtful comments drew others to him like iron filings to a magnet—their mutual stirrings, their first assignation in Dinkytown. How easy it had seemed back then, how important.

Two weeks later, they met again in Dinkytown for dinner at Vescio's, a homestyle Italian eatery known for red sauce and celebrities, sports figures like Minnesota Twins pitcher Frank Viola who ate family pasta dinners before every home game in the 1980s, an unpretentious venue favored by students and faculty. "Dinkytown is so quiet during winter break," Cate had remarked.

"You'll have to see it when it bustles."

"Is that an invitation?"

"It sure is." Jeff covered her hand with his. She turned her hand to intertwine fingers.

"When we're done eating, will you show me the rest of Dinkytown?" Cate asked.

"Sure," said Jeff, gripping her hand. She pulled at it playfully, and he squeezed before releasing it. "I've been thinking about you a lot," he said.

"Good, because I've been thinking about you," said Cate.

"For one thing, I loved your seminar."

"You want to talk about work?"

"I want to talk about *you*. That transformational stuff you teach seems like a perfect fit, and I want to know how you got interested in it."

Cate felt her cheeks grow warm. "Then I guess we can talk about work," she said. Her interest had started with Nelson Mandela, his walk to freedom in February 1990, and his address to Congress that June, around the time of high school graduation.

Then, in Cate's junior year in Aix-en-Provence, the year Mandela became president, her roommate was a white anti-apartheid South African. Cate spent the summer in Cape Town with her before heading home, a time when Mandela infused his country with inclusiveness and forgiveness. After the Springboks, an all-white rugby team won the World Cup, Mandela wore the number of the team captain to present the trophy. "He knew how to use symbolism," said Cate, and paused to laugh at herself. "God, I sound like a professor."

"You sound like you. I get that Mandela's walk to freedom was heady stuff when you were in high school, but why did it make such an impression on you?"

"Adolescence is a good time to be impressed."

"It feels more personal," said Jeff.

"I guess there was something personal about it." Cate described her miscreant, bigoted father, her charismatic, hardworking mother who respected others, who saved until she could afford a divorce. "I remember thinking that Mandela was a male figure like my mom. He filled a void."

"Sounds like your mom made her own opportunity."

"Eventually, she did. I was always interested in what made my parents so different from one another, what motivated some people to succeed, what made some people lead and others fail. As I learned about the world in college, combining psychology and business felt like a natural. My junior year abroad and summer in South Africa cemented Mandela to all of that."

"Something revved your motor enough to get into the University of Pennsylvania. I read your bio when I signed up for your seminar."

"I didn't want to be like my dad, and Mom thought an education would keep me from depending on anyone, so I worked hard, got good grades, and wrote good essays. Maybe the violin helped."

Originally, Cate wanted to play the flute, but so did every fourth-grade girl. To narrow the field, the music teacher limited the flute to girls with buckteeth; the flute was supposed to help the bite. The teacher needed violins and handed Cate a school loaner, which turned out to be a good fit. Perhaps violin was in her genes;

her uncle Eddie played violin in the St. Louis Municipal Opera. In high school, she taught violin to younger students. In her senior high school year, when they needed more violins, she played a concert with the Washington University Symphony Orchestra conducted by Leonard Slatkin.

"You had to rely on yourself," said Jeff. "I had two working parents and a peaceful home."

"Where did you go to college?"

"Harvard. Then I got my graduate degree at the U. How did you get to Aix?"

He's keeping the focus on me, Cate thought. She described her mom's remarriage to a great guy, financially secure, in her sophomore year of college, so she could afford a junior year abroad. Cate took the last sip of wine. "That's what I want for my family, calm security."

The plates and wine glasses were empty. "Didn't Bob Dylan play at the Purple Onion?" she asked, not wanting the evening to end.

"Actually, he played at a pizza joint in St. Paul with that name. It closed long ago, but the coffee shop in Dinkytown adopted its name. Dylan did play in Dinkytown at a different coffee house, the 10 O'clock Scholar."

"That's a funny name."

Jeff chuckled. "It's from Mother Goose. A nursery rhyme about a student who's always late."

"I could never be like that." Cate shook her head and laughed. "I'm always early."

"I'll bet you are." Jeff slipped his hand over hers. "Your leadership interest reminds me of Dylan. *Blowin' In the Wind* and *The Times They Are A-Changin'* are about transformation."

"Dylan's a poet and a musical genius, but I'm not sure he was making a point. He soaked up the cultural influences of his time and wrote about them."

"But the lyrics, if you listen carefully, are timeless. They could be about globalization."

Cate laughed again. "You're right about the lyrics, but I'm not Dylan. I'm a dry academic."

"There's nothing dry about you. You're fresh and exciting." His warm fingers interlocked with hers.

"I read somewhere that Dylan lived in Dinkytown," she said. "Do you know where?"

"Right across the street, that corner building with the scaffolding and the sign that says 'Future home of the Loring Pasta Bar.' You can still see the word 'Drugs' in the tile above the door. For most of the fifteen months Dylan spent in Minneapolis in 1959 and 1960, he lived above Gray's Drugs. Let's take a walk down 4th Street, and I'll show you his apartment window. It overlooks the alley."

"Positively 4th Street?"

"Some people think so. But he also hung out on 4th Street in Greenwich Village." They walked, shoulders touching, to the alley past Gray's. Jeff pointed out Dylan's window on the second floor, closest to the street. From the upstairs window of Book House, a bookstore in the building in Dinkydale across the alley, one could look directly into the window of Dylan's old room.

"I love Bob Dylan," said Cate, squeezing Jeff's hand and holding it.

"A lot happened to him in Dinkytown," said Jeff. "He heard Woody Guthrie's music, read Guthrie's book, *Bound for Glory,* switched from electric to acoustic guitar, honed his style, stopped calling himself Robert Zimmerman, and decided to go to New York."

"That's fascinating. Say, where did the name Dinkytown come from?"

"There are lots of stories about that," said Jeff, facing Cate, still holding her hand.

"I want to hear them."

"Railroad yards form one edge of Dinkytown. Small locomotives called 'dinkeys' moved rail cars around, and the chicken snacks sold in the yards were called 'dinkys.' Then there was Dinky Rog, a well-known university football player who spent time there with friends in the late 1940s."

"I love it," said Cate. "I love being here with you."

"Let's walk some more." They strolled back past the Book House to the Art Deco Varsity Theatre. "There's a lot of history here.

Imagine minstrel shows, vaudeville, comedians, and silent films, an underground club with nights of wrestling." Cate put an arm around his waist, and he reciprocated. Past the theatre marquee was the site of Marly Rusoff's bookstore and its second-story loft, where Robert Bly read poems in the early 1970s, which became a gathering place for writers and evolved into a literary center that outgrew Dinkytown. "It's called the Loft, and it just moved into new digs a mile away, on the other side of the river, but it's part of Dinkytown lore."

"What else is here?"

"I'll show you." They walked back to 14th Avenue, turned left, and looked into Al's Breakfast, a ten-foot-wide building crammed into a former alleyway across the street from Vescio's. "It looks closed," said Cate.

"It's only open for breakfast, but look inside." Cate could see fourteen stools and a yellow linoleum counter. "In the morning, there are long lines of students, artists, professors, and others who line up along the back wall, waiting for omelets and buttermilk pancakes, with a line that stretches into the street. Last May, Al's turned fifty and a brass quintet played on the sidewalk, music composed just for Al's by David Baldwin."

"I'd love to go there with you," said Cate. She removed her arm from around Jeff's waist and held his hand. He grinned and pecked her forehead.

"There's even more history on 14th Avenue," he said. "The Podium in Dylan's time sold top-of-the-line guitars. Besides Dylan, Bonnie Raitt, who recorded her first album near Minneapolis in 1971, reportedly bought guitars here. And Jerry Raskin started the Needle Doctor, right next to Al's, first selling cassettes from backpacks, until he became the go-to guy for turntable and needle repair."

"History. It's lovely," said Cate.

Jeff had grinned. "History. Maybe we could start our own."

* * *

Listening to Holst, passing the Sculpture Garden, thinking about Dinkytown, the past eleven and a half years—it made Cate cry.

Dinkytown had become a planet in their family galaxy: Pasta at Vescio's, egg rolls and Chinese at Shuang Cheng, baked goods at the Purple Onion that had modernized and moved around the corner to University Avenue, hamburgers with the kids at the McDonald's. Cate's McDonald's-owning stepfather told her that this restaurant, which ranged over two floors, was the first McDonald's in the country to gross one million dollars in a year, another fact in the lore of Dinkytown.

Cate reached the ramp at HCMC and parked. Despite all she had to do, half an hour passed before she opened the car door, plodded across Eighth Street to the hospital, and found Jeff in his recliner. Cate crossed the threshold, head still swirling, and tucked a measure of warmth into her voice. "Good morning, honey."

"Hi ... Cate." She put her arms around his shoulders and kissed him. He pushed back, head firm, lips flaccid. The soft lips unsettled her, and she withdrew to look at him, his eyes devoid of energy. Head firm, toneless kiss, eyes empty—it felt like before the accident, the way Jeff could be present and absent at the same time, nodding at her without listening, at times responding to the children in a halfhearted way that left them disappointed.

He was different from the Jeff she loved and married, the husband she'd always wanted, a contrast to her biological dad, who would listen and fade, build her hopes and thrash them. Cate had tried again and again to engage her father, but she always came away dejected. She'd understood on an intellectual level how this made her vulnerable. But now she felt this vulnerability in her bones—her father present and absent—and understood why Jeff's periods of inconstant attention enraged her.

And here was Jeff. Injured. And, despite his faults, she loved him. They had had the fight, the necessary fight, and had a chance to heal—if Jeff recovered.

Cate sat beside him, holding his hand, stroking his arm, with barely a trace of life in his eyes, and let her thoughts and feelings run. Gradually, she calmed. Although she had much to do at work, she didn't want to leave.

She checked Jeff's schedule. There was a free hour before his first visit with OT. "Jeff, let's take a walk outside this damn hospital."

"Okay," he said. "A walk."

She'd brought his down jacket from home when he moved to rehab, as if a coat in his closet would speed recovery. Without prompting, he opened his closet. Cate showed him the gloves in the pocket, and he put them on too. They walked to the elevator, marched out the front door, and circled the block. The temperature hovered just below freezing, and the day was crisp and sunny, the sidewalks clear of snow and ice, and to Cate, it felt invigorating. She wrapped an arm around Jeff's waist and remembered the walk in Dinkytown. "Jeff, put your arm around me." He looked at his arm, unsure what to do. She guided him. They finished the walk, arms around each other's waists, and returned to his room just as Kim appeared.

"Looks like you took a walk," she said.

"Walk," said Jeff. "It was cold."

"Your cheeks are rosy, and you look great. Ready for an hour in the kitchen?"

"Yes," he said and started for the door.

"I'd suggest leaving your coat in the closet," said Kim. He seemed to notice it in the mirror, removed it, and looked at it. He stood there, holding the coat, so Kim pointed to the closet, and he draped it over a hanger.

"Ready," he said.

"See you later, honey," said Cate and kissed him goodbye.

She walked to the car, her head still full, and drove to the university, collecting her thoughts.

On her desk sat a copy of the current journal article she was writing, with coauthor annotations by Jack Ross. She left it there, brewed a cup of coffee, and looked out her window, trying to make sense of all that contributed to her current reality.

* * *

When Cate looked at her watch, two hours had passed. It was almost eleven, and she was glad that no one had interrupted. Jeff's faster-than-expected progress with alertness, his returning language facility, and his deceptively normal physical appearance had encouraged her. Yet she couldn't escape the apparition of the man who looked like Jeff but wasn't Jeff.

Her thoughts turned to the children, who were hurting. She called Bonnie, the school guidance counselor and a friend.

"Good morning, Cate. I've been thinking of you. What's the latest with Jeff?"

"It's slow going. What have the kids told you?"

"Different things. Ben said he had a bad concussion and was home for Christmas but didn't want to say much more. I can tell he's worried. Kayla said he had a brain injury and isn't like his old self, and she hopes he'll get better. When I ask her how she's doing, she says she's okay, but it's hard on everybody. I sense a mix of resignation and acceptance."

"She's the resilient one."

"She's older too."

Cate heard something in the background. "Is that Sparks? It sounds like he's panting." Cate had raised the money to buy Sparks, the golden retriever guidance dog that assisted Bonnie at Eisenhower Elementary School.

"It's him. He had a run in the gym, chasing basketballs with kids who needed to let off steam."

"Nice. Glad to hear he's on his game."

"Always. Listen, I've talked with the teachers. Any chance you can stop in? I'm free for the next couple of hours."

Cate thought for a minute. She had a desk full of projects but no scheduled appointments until the afternoon. "I can get there in about a half hour, before lunch."

"Good. Sparks and I will wait for you."

* * *

Bonnie and an eager Sparks greeted Cate with hugs and licks. Cate rubbed the dog's neck. "Tell me what the children are like at home," said Bonnie.

"Same as at school. I think you nailed it when we talked before. Ben gets quiet and pulls into himself."

"It's Ben I want to talk about. Here too, he can clam up and not participate, even if the class is discussing the logic of a story or a math problem, things he's good at. It's like he's afraid his answer's not right. We see that in his homework, too; it's riddled with cross-outs and corrections."

"Does he fidget a lot in class?"

"Mostly tapping, in beats of two."

"That's Ben. Perfectionism and tapping."

"You've clearly thought about it. What do you think is going on?"

"My sister, Copper, has OCD."

"When I discussed Ben's behaviors with the school psychologist, he mentioned the possibility of OCD and suggested a child psychiatrist and a therapist."

"Copper talked to Ben about her OCD, which I think helped because he likes her. She's fun, and it seemed to ease his anxiety when she named it. She made the same recommendations to us, but I haven't called anybody."

"I'd get started. There's a shortage of child psychiatrists, and appointments are hard to get."

"His pediatrician should have some ideas," said Cate.

"Good. Remember that Sparks makes house calls," said Bonnie. "He's been known to make weekend visits."

Cate chuckled. "The kids would like that. We all would when things settle down a bit."

On the drive back to the university, Cate called the pediatrician and reached the nurse. She said that primary care had a relationship with mental health. She called mental health intake, gave Cate the number, and suggested that she call them in fifteen minutes. Therapy was easier to schedule than psychiatry. As Cate walked from the ramp to her office, she scheduled the first available therapy appointment in eighteen days, on a Monday, the day that her symposium ended.

* * *

As full and emotional as the day had been, the symposium rose to the top of Cate's priorities. She wanted to check on conference details and had scheduled an hour with Jennifer. After that, she wanted to review her keynote yet again, although she could remember every slide, every nuance, even the jokes and when to insert them. Then she had a meeting with Rosie, always a bright spot in her day; they'd review Rosie's plans for the breakout session. Cate had scheduled two short meetings with other graduate students to end the day. Shepherding students toward doctorates, nurturing them, was the most gratifying part of Cate's job.

Her meetings went well. Jennifer promised to arrive early at the Convention Center on the first day of the symposium to make sure everything ran smoothly. That way, Cate could have breakfast with the kids and get to the conference in plenty of time for her keynote.

Rosie had prepared thoughtful comments to introduce the breakout seminar and described how she might shape the conversation depending on what attendees brought to the discussion. *I'm going to enjoy watching this,* Cate thought. Two meetings later, and she was out the door.

CHAPTER TWENTY-EIGHT:

Symposium, January 18-21

Cate awoke energized on Friday morning. She got the kids off to school, called Jeff so he could hear her voice, and headed for the Minneapolis Convention Center. A year of preparation would culminate today.

Promptly at nine, Jennifer stood, welcomed the registrants, and introduced Cate as the primary organizer and keynote speaker of the conference. Cate thanked her, made a few welcoming remarks, and said she was excited to talk about transformational leadership.

Thoughts of Jeff lingered beneath the surface. He had listened many times to her keynote and helped her shape it.

"I'd like to begin with a question about individuals. What qualities of character make some individuals succeed and others fail?" Cate asked. "Please shout out some answers."

The audience responded. Values. The capacity to adapt. Resilience.

"Yes, and the same qualities apply to family businesses, not-for-profits, corporations in a global economy, and civilizations. When I was in high school in 1990, Mandela walked to freedom. We think of him as a transformational leader. Was he?" Heads nodded. "I agree, but why? Shout it out."

Vision.

"Yes. Mandela wanted an inclusive multiracial society."

Forgiveness.

"Yes, again. Perpetrators could acknowledge misdeeds before Bishop Desmond Tutu's Truth and Reconciliation Commission.

Generosity.

"Agree. Mandela did not want a nation filled with angry, demoralized Afrikaners."

"These are the qualities of transformational leaders. In the business world, we think of Jack Welch at General Electric as a transformational leader. Was he?"

Jeff had suggested this question.

Some thought yes, but there were murmurs of hesitation. Welch had sold off major divisions and slashed GE's size to position it for growth.

"I understand the dissent. Perhaps we can agree that the first part of GE's transformation was difficult but essential. Then Jack Welch hired Noel Tichy. In a 1989 article, one year before Mandela's walk to freedom, Tichy argued that change was hard, that leaders had to acknowledge loss and care for everyone in the best way possible, that respect for individuals was fundamental. Autonomy was the essential ingredient for innovation. By appointing Tichy to head GE's leadership center, Welch implemented that vision. Many think hiring Tichy was Welch's best decision."

"I understand the general idea," said one attendee, "but how does it work?"

"Perfect question." Cate said that she and her faculty had designed the entire symposium to address that issue, with plenary addresses and breakout sessions.

"This is personal to me."

Personal. The idea of making the symposium personal was Jeff's. Cate struggled to maintain composure. She would need all her leadership skills, all the qualities she had just described, to rebuild her life, to adapt to Jeff's injury.

"In my family, some individuals thrived, and others stagnated or declined, and I wanted to know why. Mandela inspired me. Learning about Welch and Tichy informed me. Let's make this weekend personal for you."

When she finished, Jennifer returned to the podium. "You've just seen Cate model the kind of leadership we're talking about." A small crowd gathered beneath the stage, and Cate descended the stairs for more discussion. After the crowd dispersed, Jennifer spoke to Cate.

"If you need to visit Jeff, it's okay to leave."

"You know I made arrangements to stay, and he's fine."

"I just thought ..."

"Look, Jennifer, I appreciate the nice things you said, but your offer doesn't feel right. If you're thinking about anything, it's yourself." Anger at Jennifer had been smoldering. "We're talking about leadership and character here, so please lose the bullshit." She turned her back and left.

* * *

On Saturday morning, Jack delivered his plenary address with panache, his thick brown eyebrows in constant motion above hazel eyes, his face animated, his beard well-trimmed and longer on the chin, his red necktie braided into a perfect half Windsor, dapper in a gray Harris Tweed suit. He described the way that culture, Asian or Western, is built into the DNA of international companies. Culture affects how global companies view each other and how they compete. Then he described his plans to collaborate with Japanese scholars at Fukushima University to study why the Fukushima earthquake and tsunami surprised business, government, and the surrounding community, to see if culture played a role.

Cate loved the way Jack galvanized the room. She beamed when he cited their paper about business and national culture and credited her. When the post-lecture discussion concluded, there was barely time for a collegial hug before Jack left for the airport.

"Take care, and I'll see you in March, but there's always the phone," he said. "I'll be thinking of you and Jeff."

To Cate's delight, Jack waved at Jennifer but offered no hug. As she and Jennifer reviewed summaries prepared by leaders of yesterday's breakout seminars, Jennifer, quiet and contrite, made no attempt at small talk.

In midafternoon, after a quick call to say hi to Jeff, Cate arrived at the breakout seminar that Rosie would lead, and watched Rosie bring the meeting to order. The seminar examined the psychological stress that leaders feel in times of turmoil and how they deal with it. "Picture two CEOs, one with walled-off emotion, one who acknowledges stress to himself and seeks support from colleagues, friends, and family," said Rosie. They examined what it felt like to work in organizations whose leaders had such different styles and how that affected resilience and success. How do these styles affect direct reports, and how do they percolate through leadership ranks to everyone?

It was a pleasure for Cate to watch Rosie work. Although a conference on transformational leadership might seem to favor softer, more aware leaders, Rosie didn't allow easy conclusions. She probed ideas, generated questions, provoked discussion, and in a respectful way, challenged responses. *Twelve years ago, the day I met Jeff, that was me,* Cate thought.

On Monday, feeling elated, Cate began her summation, which Jeff had helped her compose. "In what ways are leaders affected by their personal history and values? By the cultures of their nations and organizations? How do leaders consider these issues in guiding transformational change? Respecting individuals? Promoting innovation? If you're thinking about these issues in a new way, this conference has succeeded."

Precisely at noon, Cate ended the conference.

CHAPTER TWENTY-NINE:

Monday afternoon, Hospital Day 50, January 21

Immediately after the symposium, Cate, Jennifer, and Rosie met at The Local in downtown Minneapolis for lunch and celebration. Jennifer offered a toast to Cate, who toasted Jennifer in return. They both praised Rosie, whom they'd asked to edit the written Proceedings, the published record of the exciting weekend. The decision pleased Cate: earlier than most, Rosie had begun the transition from student to colleague.

As Cate ate vegetarian curry and sipped a diet Coke, eschewing beer, she sat with her head in the clouds, yet her feet grew heavy. After an hour of merriment, Cate made a joke about diving back into motherhood and marriage and departed for Eisenhower Elementary.

She reached the school at half past one, planning to meet Bonnie for an update on both kids, observe Ben, and take Ben to his therapy appointment at three. Bonnie greeted her, and Sparks put his paws on Cate's lap and gazed into her eyes with a soft whimper. Bonnie smiled. "Sparks thinks you need to chill. He knows you have to finish with one world before you enter another."

"Sparks is a smart dog. It does feel like an abrupt transition."

"We'd love to hear about the symposium, wouldn't we, Sparks?" The dog gave an encouraging woof and crawled up next to Cate, who hesitated and glanced at her watch. "There's plenty of time," said Bonnie. "Chatting with us will help Ben a lot more than charging into his room for two minutes of observation and scooping him into the arms of a therapist."

Cate laughed. "I guess that's my style, charging from one thing to another, but it does sound absurd when you put it that way." Cate described the symposium's high points, chatting for ten minutes as Sparks listened, head cocked, eyes alert. Cate rubbed his neck, enjoying the physical contact, and felt her tension ease. "You're right about changing worlds. I'm almost ready. She looked up, and Bonnie was smiling.

"This is the first time you've seen Sparks the guidance dog in action. You gave him to us, but you've never felt his gentle power."

"He's awesome. The two of you make a great team."

"This team makes tea, don't we, Sparks?" Sparks curled his lips into a dog smile, wagged his tail, and yipped. Bonnie brewed two cups of chamomile tea with water from an electric pot and filled Sparks' bowl with cool water. Cate and Bonnie and Sparks sipped.

"I can see why all the kids love you," Cate said.

"Guiding kids and parents is part of the job, but lunch is about friendship. Pull out your calendar and let's set a date." They found one in a couple of weeks. "Now we're ready to talk about the kids. To start with, tell me in more detail what you see at home, especially with Ben."

Cate thought about the answer. She'd made it a point, despite the busy weekend, to spend time with the children every morning and evening. "Ben's worries vary in severity, but he gets sick to his stomach almost every morning. You already know about his habits. Kayla takes charge of things, which seems to work for her. It's her way of staying in control."

"I think you're right. Kayla told her class about her dad's injury and was able to say that she's sad and worried but liked his Christmas visit. She seems mature and resilient."

"That's Kayla."

"Ben gave his teacher permission to tell his class about his dad's injury but won't talk about it himself, even when other kids approach him. He's always been a popular kid. That helps. Regarding homework, he's doing better at getting it done, but never thinks it's good enough. I asked Ben, and he said it's okay for us to visit his classroom. Ben and his teacher expect us."

"Poor Ben. I'm glad he has a therapy appointment."

"You told me it's with June Hatwig?"

"Yes."

"Good, I've worked with her before, and kids like her. She does a good job coordinating with school so we're all on the same page." Bonnie asked Cate to sign a release so that June and she could communicate and gave her a copy to give to June. Sparks sat up, wagging his tail. "I guess it's time to go," said Bonnie.

They walked to Ben's classroom and stood quietly in the doorway. Ben was seated in a far corner of the room with his back to the door, working on a project with a girl Cate recognized as his friend Jill. Except for an occasional two-tap, Ben seemed okay. All the kids sat in groups around the room. The teacher saw Cate and Bonnie, walked to the door, and whispered. "Ben's working on a Science Buddies STEM project about simple machines," she whispered, "an approach we use in third grade for our brightest kids. This one is about levers." Arrayed around Ben and his classmate were books of different weights, a rod to act as a fulcrum, rulers of various lengths, and a felt pen to mark the rulers. To figure out how to lift a book with one finger, the students had to plan investigations, identify variables, gather and record data, and work collaboratively. "Watch for a while, see how they plan and mark the rulers, and I'll be back." Ben managed to stay on task, except that his two-taps increased each time an experiment failed; once, he stood up and did several jumping jacks while his partner worked. His classmate seemed unperturbed by his nervousness.

Ben still had his back to the doorway when the teacher returned. "You can see Ben's anxiety, but this is a good day, probably because his mind is engaged, and Jill is a good partner for him. Actually, she reminds me of Kayla. Maybe that's why they like each other. If we're working as a class, not in small groups, he shakes and can't get the answer out when I call on him." Cate shook her head. Sparks rubbed against her legs.

"You can see how he gets upset when something doesn't work, with those two-taps and jumping jacks," said Bonnie. The teacher agreed and mentioned his homework with all the cross-outs. Even working on assignments in class, he reviews his work so many times that he wears himself out.

"If it helps, I've seen this twice before," said Bonnie. "Both kids got better enough to function normally."

"I taught one of them," said the teacher.

"Do either of you think Ben has OCD?"

"That's making a diagnosis, which we can't do," said Bonnie, "but I can tell you the two kids I mentioned had OCD, and you told me about your sister, Copper. Cate, whatever you call it, he's a kid who's hurting."

"You're right. He's a sensitive kid, and we're all under stress."

It was time to end the project, and the teacher pointed Ben toward his mom; he hurried to her side as Sparks woofed a friendly greeting. Once they were in the hallway, out of sight of the class, Ben flew into his mother's arms. Cate hugged him until his grip relaxed.

"What were you working on?" she asked.

"Levers. We were scientists figuring stuff out."

"It looked like fun."

"Jill's my favorite partner. She's smart, and it doesn't bother her when I get worried."

"It's nice to have a good comrade."

They said goodbye to Bonnie. Ben fetched his coat from the hall locker, and they walked to the car. On the drive, Ben was quiet until Cate engaged him, then he asked several questions about his appointment. Cate said June was someone he could talk to about his worries, even getting sick in the morning. "Will she stop the worries, Mommy?"

"She'll help you understand them, so they don't bother you as much, like Aunt Copper does with her worries."

"You mean figure them out, like the lever?"

"Kind of, but it's not like putting marks on rulers."

"I don't want my worries to scare her."

"They won't, honey. She's used to kids with worries.

* * *

At the clinic, June smiled as she stepped into the waiting room and introduced herself. "Hi, Ben, it's nice to meet you. Bring your mom and come on in." Ben peeked into the office and hesitated at the door, clinging to his mother.

"Don't you have a dog?" he asked.

"I have a dog at home, a boxer named Zeus."

Ben looked disappointed.

"Bet you're thinking of Sparks. I've met him, Bonnie too, when I visited your school."

That brought a grin to Ben's face. He released his mom's arm and followed June into the office. "Ben, I'd like to hear why you came to see me."

"My worries." He started to two-tap, fingers against his thigh.

"When your mom made this appointment, she said your dad had an accident. Is that right?" The two-taps accelerated into a constant rhythm.

"Yeah. He hurt his head and he's in the hospital, but he visited us on Christmas."

"When did you see him last?"

"This weekend. Grandma and Grandpa took us while Mom was at her work thing. He knew us better than before."

"He didn't always know you?"

"Now he does."

"I see. When's he coming home for good?"

"In a few weeks, when he's better. I miss him." To Cate's relief, Ben seemed to like June and talked easily. His two-taps slowed.

"I'm sure you do. Ben, since this is our first appointment, I would like to visit with your mom for twenty minutes or so, then just with you, and at the end with both of you. Would you mind hanging out in the waiting room while I talk to your mom?" Ben looked back and forth between June and his mom.

"Can I read? I have a book in my backpack."

"Sure. What's the book about?"

"Jack Stalwart." He opened his backpack and showed it to her. "I just started it, but it's about Jack finding his brother in Egypt."

"I like that one. I've read all the Jack Stalwart books to my kids at home."

"You have?" The two-taps stopped.

"Yes." She smiled and Ben grinned in return. June held the door open, and he exited to the waiting room.

"He seems like a good kid with a lot to handle," said June. "How are you holding up?"

"It's been tough." Cate briefly described Jeff's injury, his progress to date and uncertain prognosis, the kids' visits to the hospital, the Christmas visit, and how both kids were responding, especially Ben's worries and behavior at home and school. Although Ben had always been anxious, these problems were new. She told June about Copper's OCD and her discussion with Ben.

"Ben said something about your symposium." In as few words as possible, Cate described the weekend, her work at the university, and clarified that she was an organizational psychologist, not a clinical psychologist.

"You're a busy person. There's a lot on your shoulders."

"I can't think about that. I just keep moving forward, grateful to have lots of support from friends and family. The kids do too." She told June about her uptight nature, that Jeff was more easygoing. June asked about the marriage and Cate described the marital tension but did not think it affected Ben and Kayla, who had good relationships with both parents before the accident. She described Jeff's background and achievements.

Cate liked June's easy manner.

She held the door ajar as Cate left, and Ben, with a brief glance at his mom, disappeared into her office. Cate stared at a magazine, unable to think about anything except Ben, hoping June could help. When June opened the door again, Ben looked at ease, curled into a chair in June's office.

"Do you want to tell your mom what we think, or should I?" asked June.

"I'm scared about Daddy. Suppose he doesn't get better and doesn't come home." Ben teared up, and Cate hugged him.

"It's okay, sweetie. We're all worried about Dad. I wish we knew for certain that he'll get back to normal, but I promise he'll get better enough to come home from the hospital."

"June says getting sick in the morning is part of my worries." He looked at June and seemed to gain confidence. "We think I have OCD like Aunt Copper, and I can do really well like Aunt Copper."

"Looks like all of us have the same idea," said Cate.

"June says learning to live with OCD is like solving a puzzle. If I figure out what's happening, like my two-taps, I can learn to let go so they don't bother me," said Ben.

"Do you know what letting go means?" asked June.

"Not yet, but you said I'd figure that out. You said it might take time, but it's not too hard."

Cate laughed, relieved by Ben's optimism and trust. Ben liked puzzles and Cate could tell that he liked June, who recommended weekly puzzle-solving visits for two months. Then they could evaluate progress.

"Do you think Ben is depressed?" asked Cate.

"Maybe. Ben and I talked about that too. It's pretty common with OCD. Even without depression, a medication like Prozac is what we recommend for OCD." She had asked mental health intake to hold an appointment with a child psychiatrist on Friday, which Cate, with agreement from Ben, accepted.

June leaned forward. "Cate, a diagnosis is just a way of thinking about Ben's symptoms, even if a name makes you more secure and suggests the use of medication. He's a kid with real-life stress who's scared. That's our focus. That's what Ben and I discussed."

CHAPTER THIRTY:

Tuesday, Hospital Day 51, January 22

At breakfast, Cate chatted with the children. The forecast of snow, lots of it, excited them all, and the kids wanted to talk about outdoor activities for the weekend, even though it was four days away. They had heard on TV that conditions, thick powder, not too cold, would be ideal for skiing and snowboarding. Ben had asked for and received a snowboard, which Jeff had helped unwrap on Christmas day.

"Evie told me there's cross-country skiing at the Arboretum," said Kayla. "They ski and study trees in winter."

"If we're gonna ski instead of snowboard, I'd rather downhill." Ben, who was athletic like both parents, could navigate green circle and even some blue square trails.

Kayla looked up from her cell phone. "I checked. The cross-country stuff at the Arboretum is Saturday. We could do that, then snowboard and downhill at Hyland Hills on Sunday after gymnastics. Ben, you could bring your new snowboard and your skis to Hyland."

"Cool!" said Ben. "Specially if David comes."

"We could all go," said Kayla. She looked at Jeff's empty chair. "You know, moms and kids."

"Good idea. I'll call Meg," said Cate. "Hey, the clock says it's almost time for school."

Like a switch had flipped, Ben grew pale and retched. Cate thought about her conversation with Copper early that morning. "Ben, it's okay; we're going to help you with your worries."

"I'm scared about Dad too, Ben, but I talk about it. You show it with your worries," said Kayla.

"Thanks, honey! What do you think about that, big guy?"

"I don't know," said Ben, but he zipped up his backpack without repacking it, reached for his sister's hand, and squeezed it as color returned to his face.

The children donned coats and waited on the brick steps with the front door partially open, allowing heat from the house to warm their backs. When the bus pulled into sight, they ran past the snow family and climbed aboard. Cate, from the stoop, watched them round the corner, thinking about Ben's worries and Kayla's wisdom.

Cate closed the door, and at once, the pressures of the day ahead burgeoned. She enjoyed a tension-relieving shower massage and drove to the hospital, remembering to bring a dress shirt from home, a blue tattersall that Jeff loved. Kim in OT wanted Jeff to work on buttons.

Kim was already there when Cate arrived. Jeff grinned when he saw the shirt, as if it were familiar. He put one arm through a sleeve, then the other, but the shirt and cuffs hung open. Kim showed him a button and the matching buttonhole, but he seemed uncertain how to proceed. "What do you want to do?" asked Kim.

"Put on the shirt."

"Here's what you'll do." She showed him how to grasp the front of his shirt, expose a hole, grasp the opposing button with the other hand, and push it through. After help with a few buttons, he finished the front on his own but needed help with the cuffs. Kim asked him to button and unbutton the cuffs a couple of times, which he did with difficulty. "You're making progress, Jeff. We'll practice that again this afternoon or tomorrow." She smiled at Cate and Jeff and left.

Cate checked the schedule. "You're done with OT; now it's time for Rudy."

"Speech and lang…widge."

"That's right, honey." An aide arrived to direct him, but Cate said she'd take him. With prompting from Cate, Jeff was able to find Rudy's office.

"Welcome," said Rudy. "Jeff, do you remember that this is our last session? This is your graduation day."

"I remember."

"You're doing very well. Even though you still have a little difficulty saying what you want, that will improve without therapy. If you feel stuck, or Cate thinks more treatment might help, you can always call me, but in another month, I'll bet you'll be speaking normally. Maybe an occasional problem finding just the right word. Do you understand?"

"I'm done. Finished."

"You got it. Conversation is important, so use your language whenever you can. It's like exercising your body. You have to keep at it."

"Thank you. Umm, g'bye," said Jeff. Rudy patted his shoulder.

"Rudy, you've been a delight," said Cate and gave him a hug. Jeff approached Rudy, touched his arm, and, like a little boy, rested his head on Rudy's shoulder.

* * *

Back in his room, Jeff settled into his recliner and said little. "Would you like to hear about my symposium? You had good ideas when I was planning it." Jeff seemed attentive, perhaps because Cate spoke with enthusiasm. "For the welcoming banquet, we assigned seats so that people of different backgrounds sat together. You liked that idea, do you remember?"

"No."

"I wanted chief executives to sit with students. You suggested that colleagues from different countries sit together."

"To know the other."

"Yes, it was a good idea, and it worked."

"I liked it."

"You did. Do you remember Rosie?"

"Mandy," he said.

"That's right, Mandy's sister and my graduate student. She ran a seminar and did a great job."

"Hilton."

Cate sat up. "You're thinking about when we met? At my seminar?" Whatever connection Jeff had made did not persist. He looked toward the TV, at the blank screen, and yawned. "Jeff, no TV. Tell me how you're feeling?"

"Tired."

"What makes you tired?"

"I don't know."

"You get tired because you had a brain injury and thinking takes effort." Jeff stared at her. "Honey, tell me again. What happened to you?"

"Brain hurt." He looked away, frowning.

"I know. Talking wears you out and makes you anxious." Cate had left a six-pack of diet cream soda on top of his chest of drawers. She fetched ice and poured some into a cup. The familiar taste, and lack of effort, made Jeff relax.

Cate stayed through lunch and left for a quiet hour at home before the school bus arrived. Jeff's parents would visit that afternoon.

That night, after dinner and cleanup, Karen and Dan left for Northfield. Cate sent the kids to pick out books; they'd each received several for Christmas. Kayla returned with *The Birchbark House* by Louise Erdrich. Ben chose *Watership Down,* which his dad had started to read to him before the accident. Although Ben was an advanced reader, he found some of the language hard, but he dug into it and, from time to time, asked Cate for help. They read until Cate tucked them into the bunks in Kayla's room.

"Mommy, when Dad comes home, I'm gonna read *Watership Down* to him."

"I can help if you get stuck," said Kayla.

"Dad will love that," said Cate. "Good night, my sweets.

CHAPTER THIRTY-ONE:

Friday, Hospital Day 54, January 25

Cate awoke in a good mood. The kids were coping, Jeff was making progress, work was challenging and congenial, and she was handling her crazy schedule. For lunch, she and Jeff's parents had arranged a pass for Jeff to enjoy a nice restaurant away from the hospital. Cate began the day at home, drinking black tea and reading journals, looking forward to lunch and the change of pace.

She'd made good progress by the time an iPhone chime alerted her to an email from Jack Ross. He was still on sabbatical in Japan, but had a copy of their article-in-progress, annotated for revision, asking for a response within a week. Cate felt anxious and knew it was not the deadline. This was Jack's first extended trip without Liz, and a thought surprised and disconcerted her. Part of her wanted Jack to feel lonely. She read the rest of what he sent, which asked how she and Jeff and the kids were doing.

She left the computer, brewed another cup of black tea, cleared her head, and wrote a bland response, "Hope you're finding time to enjoy your lovely surroundings." Then she opened the attachment and buried herself in revision, missing the companionship of working in person. She finished her response quickly and sent it back, joking that it didn't take her a week. She'd beaten another deadline; Jack loved to tease her about not respecting deadlines. She always finished far ahead of them.

As she drove to the hospital, Cate called Jeff's parents, who met her at the door with Jeff zipped into his winter parka. They headed to Fika, which in Swedish meant "break," a fifteen-minute drive from HCMC. The restaurant, known for open-faced Nordic sandwiches and Swedish small plates, inhabited a modern space appended to an early-twentieth-century mansion that housed the American Swedish Institute, a museum and cultural center in south Minneapolis. They paused in the parking lot, savoring the crisp air, swallowing the chill. "My face is cold, but shivery and good," said Jeff. In the entryway, sumptuous smells greeted them. A small museum store opened to the right; to the left were waited tables and a cafeteria. Straight ahead, large windows opened to snow-covered tables in a spacious patio.

The Fika menu emphasized color and flavor. A waiter passed the table carrying the meatball small plate, and Cate pointed out the red lingonberry sauce, mustard, and cucumbers.

"Cucumbers and lingonberries," said Jeff. Cate smiled and ordered two, one for her and one for Jeff. Dan ordered a seared salmon sandwich, and Karen had a roasted squash salad. Only Dan had the house-made aquavit. They ordered malted meringue with chocolate, banana, and hazelnuts to share for dessert, and Cate brought cardamom bread pudding to bring home to the kids.

"We can all come back in the summer and sit on the patio," said Cate. Jeff walked to the windows that overlooked the patio and tried the door.

"It's locked," he said. "And there's snow."

"There won't be snow in the summer, honey."

After lunch, Cate dropped Jeff and his parents at the hospital door, giving Jeff a warm hug and a kiss on his flaccid lips, and headed to the university. She liked her office. Pictures and mementos created continuity, reminding her of Jeff and the children. Cate had always wanted home and work to flow together as integrated parts of her life.

Six years ago, to celebrate her promotion to associate professor and the achievement of academic tenure, Jeff had given her a wine-red Herman Miller executive chair with a bottle of 2006 Château Angelus Saint-Emilion Grand Cru taped to the seat. The empty bottle rested on a bookshelf next to a picture of Jeff cradling Kayla at three months, beaming at his daughter with enough love and pride to make the picture glow. She loved to sit at her desk, embraced by the chair, warmed by her surroundings.

Yet for the past year, especially since the accident, her office had become an escape, and the chair did not always comfort. Cate spent two busy hours working in the chair that Jeff had given her before she returned to the hospital.

As she approached Jeff's room, Cate heard the soft voices of Karen and Dan and paused outside the doorway, reminded of the time they described Jeff feeling distant from her. This time, the voices were admiring new photos taped to the wall that morning. Cate entered with a smile and asked about the pictures. In one of them, Kayla and Ben stood in front of the Christmas tree they helped to decorate, a final photo before they tossed the tree. In another, Cate and the kids stood in front of the snow family and the spirit bear on Christmas day.

Every time it snowed, Grandma helped them repair the melting that occurred when the temperature climbed above freezing.

Cate felt especially drawn to a third picture, taken last summer, of Ben pitching at an empty diamond at Big Willow Park with Jeff supervising and Kayla, Cate, and Karen watching. "Dan, you took that one," said Cate. "Remember, Jeff signed Ben up for tee ball, and he hated it; he watched older kids pitch and started practicing windups. Jeff said he'd show Ben how to pitch, but he couldn't do it until he was good enough to help his team."

"Teamwork," said Dan, thumping his chest. "I taught that to Jeff, and he passed it on."

"Give it a rest, Dan," said Karen.

"But it's important," said Dan. "Growing kids need their father."

"They do," said Cate. "They need you too, Dan—especially now."

"What they need is a grandfather, not a teacher or another doctor," said Karen with a good-humored smile. Dan had a habit of holding

Jeff's wrist as if he were checking his pulse. "I think you play doctor to reassure yourself." Dan shot her an exaggerated scowl and laughed.

That's how they do it, thought Cate. That's how they keep going.

"Cate, I never told you that Jeff called me that first evening after you met. He couldn't stop talking about you. I could tell from his voice that he was smitten even before he told me you were very attractive."

"I was smitten too."

Jeff arrived from OT, accompanied by an aide. Cate greeted him with a hug.

"Honey, do you remember that I have a meeting with Robin, the TBI social worker, this afternoon?" asked Cate. He did not. Robin wanted to schedule a home assessment and plan an overnight visit before discharge. "After that meeting, I have to leave, but I'll be back with the kids tomorrow. Your parents, too, they're staying with us for the weekend."

Cate took Jeff's hand in hers. "See you tomorrow, honey." She hugged Jeff tightly, holding on for several seconds, and kissed him on the lips. He pressed his lips against hers, a Jeff kiss with sagging lips.

* * *

"Mommy, when is Daddy coming home?" asked Ben that evening.

"In about two weeks. That's what the doctors said today."

"Really?" said Kayla, clapping her hands.

"A couple of nights before that, he'll have an overnight visit."

"Why a visit, Mom?" asked Kayla.

"It makes it easier for all of us to adjust. Then he'll be home for good."

"Will Daddy be all better when he comes home?" asked Ben.

"That's going to take a long time, sweetie."

"He promised to take me to a farm and show me how he puts embryos into cows," said Ben.

"Maybe Bill, dad's partner, can show you. I'll ask him." Cate took Ben's chin in her hands and kissed his forehead.

"I know what will help Dad get better. He likes music," said Ben.

"Mozart is Dad's favorite composer," said Kayla. They had discussed what Dad liked, what would help him feel good once he came home. The kids had selected three Mozart CDs, one Brahms and one Beethoven CD. Cate had chosen Holst's *The Planets*.

CHAPTER THIRTY-TWO:

Tuesday to Thursday, Hospital Days 58–60, January 29–31

"How can I sleep if I'm not sure he's in the best place?" With discharge to outpatient care on the horizon, Cate wanted to consider other programs besides Knapp. Meg and Karen suggested exploring the TBI program Sister Kenny.

"Both programs are excellent," said Dan, "and the program won't make a damn bit of difference to Jeff's recovery. It all depends on his injury."

Eight weeks after Jeff's accident, Cate and Jeff's parents met with Emmie Rose, the social worker, and Dr. Marie Janiscek, the rehabilitation medicine physician, at Sister Kenny. Both had good things to say about Knapp and suggested that Cate choose the place that felt most comfortable. Sister Kenny looked and felt a lot like Knapp.

"I wish Jeff could decide," said Cate. "It's his life."

"I do too, but he can't. We'll support whatever decision you make," said Karen. Dan agreed. "What does your gut say?" asked Karen.

"That's exactly what Jeff would ask," said Cate. Outside, in the snow-covered courtyard, arms lifted toward the sky drew her attention.

Cate donned her coat and, with Jeff's parents following, approached a family cast in bronze. A plaque identified the sculpture as *Wellspring,* by Paul T. Granlund. "This is a lovely piece. Do you know him, Karen?"

"Sure, I did a workshop with Granlund. His compositions suggest hope and spirituality, so a lot of his work resides at hospitals and churches. The Arboretum is building a new sculpture garden, and he'll be there too."

"The Arboretum? Maybe that's a sign," said Cate.

* * *

The next morning, Robin, the Knapp social worker, conducted the predischarge home assessment and found no physical barriers. Although Jeff could manage stairs, bathroom tasks, and simple kitchen tasks like eating cold cereal with milk, he would need supervision using sharp objects or preparing hot food. Cate might want to choose his clothes, at least for a while, so they'd match. With 24/7 supervision, he wouldn't harm himself or wander outside.

After the inspection, Robin and Cate sipped tea on the four-season porch. "What arrangements have you made for discharge?" asked Robin.

"My sister will be here for the first week. After that, we have our nanny, friends, family, a retired neighbor for transportation to outpatient rehab, and the agency you recommended as backup." Cate hesitated, then asked what she thought about Sister Kenny.

"Are you thinking of going there instead of Knapp?" asked Robin with a knowing smile.

"Maybe. Not that I don't appreciate all that HCMC and Knapp have done."

"But making a change feels like you're taking charge?"

"Yes. How did you know?"

"I've been doing this for a long time, and I understand the appeal of a fresh start. My only concern is your expectations. His injury and not the program will determine his prognosis."

"Jeff's dad agrees."

"If that's what you decide, I'll be glad to facilitate transfer of his records. But you have to promise to let us know how he's doing."

"Thanks. You couldn't be more gracious."

In the garden, evergreens, bushes, and two leafless oaks rose above the snow, and beyond the split rail fence, maples and ashes punctuated the rolling hills. The view was pastoral but didn't match Cate's apprehension.

"I can see you're worried," said Robin. "Discharge is a big step and a big adjustment." She patted Cate's arm. "The other thing we have to discuss is finances. That's a constant worry for families in your situation." Cate nodded. Money was tight, despite Cate's income. Jeff's disability policy provided a fraction of the salary he'd drawn from his business, and expenses were rising. After a year of disability, she recommended that Jeff apply for Social Security, and Jeff had long-term-care insurance.

On the other side of the ledger, personal expenses had increased. The first hospital bill had arrived, and the amount was staggering—over $250,000, and the claim against the driver of the other car was far from settled. Jeff's health insurance company had begun to question some of the rehab therapies with the prior authorization process, and that might get worse with outpatient care. After discharge, expenses would include the agency that helped provide 24/7 supervision, which long-term insurance might cover.

"I've talked with other families," said Cate. "Hard as it is for us, we're damn lucky with our resources."

"That's true," said Robin. "Some folks with TBI, especially when it isn't from an accident, end up on Medicaid."

"I know this isn't kind, but I wish the driver of the other car was alive and struggling with all of this," said Cate.

"You don't need to apologize. It can feel like you got the worst of it."

On the crest of a distant hill, a deer loped, joined by a larger deer with a short neck, probably a male that had recently shed its antlers. They stood together, two sleek animals with gray-brown winter coats. Jeff had told the children that bucks grow new antlers every spring;

by midsummer, one could discern the shape of the new rack. Cate wondered what Jeff would be like in midsummer. It seemed so far away.

"Let's talk about Jeff's overnight pass," said Robin. "The team thought we could aim for a week from today, which would be a Wednesday. If everything goes well, he could come home that Friday."

"I can have help next Wednesday and throughout the weekend to make sure it goes smoothly."

"Think of Wednesday as a dress rehearsal for coming home."

"A dress rehearsal?" said Cate. She winced, and tears streamed down her cheeks. "That sounds like a play, imitating life."

Robin responded with a comforting smile. "Transitions can be scary, especially this one. A dress rehearsal can identify pitfalls and make discharge easier, and I use that term with intention. Theatre helps you contemplate a different reality; it lets you empathize with someone else's experience and with your own."

They continued to sip tea until Robin had to leave.

Cate promised again to stay in touch during the next several months, even if he moved to Sister Kenny.

CHAPTER THIRTY-THREE:

Monday, Hospital Day 64, February 4

Five days later, at eight in the morning, 10:00 p.m. in Japan, Cate phoned Jack from her university office for an arranged call to discuss the final draft of their journal article. Jack picked up promptly. "Hey, it's good to talk to you."

"How's Fukushima?"

"Freezing and snowing. I could be in Minneapolis, except that I'm living in a Japanese guesthouse and just spent a long evening with friends. I'm full of Fukushima dumplings called *enban gyoza.* They're filled with pork or vegetables, then baked and served crispy on a circular dish. You'd love them."

"Sounds delicious. You're always teaching me something."

"Not every evening is like that. Last night I settled for ramenburgers in a restaurant beneath the bullet train station."

"Alone?"

"Unfortunately. If Liz were here, we'd be dining out every night, studying Fukushima history, enjoying castles and scenery, and exploring the countryside—which, by the way, is beautiful. I have lots of time to look around."

"There must be a lot to see. You've told me in the past that Fukushima is full of history."

"The Boshin Civil War started here, the war that ended the feudal shogunate, unified Japan, and abolished the samurai warrior class."

Cate laughed. "That wraps Japanese history into a tight package."

"It's relevant to what we study. What started the war was exposure to other cultures, which disrupted the feudal shogunate. Today, that exposure happens with global competition."

"That is interesting." Cate spoke in a voice too honeyed. "I've learned a lot, and we've only been talking for a few minutes."

"Okay, I deserve that."

"Jack, there's a photograph in your office of a castle with lovely fall foliage. Isn't that in Fukushima?"

"It is. I took that picture of the Tsuruga-jo castle in early October when I visited for a few days to organize the sabbatical. Now it's a broad white tower with red tiles that soars above the snow. I'm told that it's surrounded by cherry blossoms in the spring."

"Then it's always lovely. Maybe I can visit sometime."

"That would make it even lovelier." Jack's voice had a touch of sadness. "How are you and the kids doing, and Jeff?"

"Jeff's coming home for an overnight pass on Wednesday and probably for good on Friday."

"That's wonderful! A big change for everyone."

"It's a milestone." Cate, on the verge of tears, paused to gather her thoughts. "He needs round-the-clock supervision, which underscores the severity of his injury. Whatever you want to call it—liveliness, energy, moxie, gumption—it's not there. It hurts like hell to see him that way."

"What do you think it's like for Jeff?"

"They say his brain has to reassemble his world, real and emotional, from fragments of perception and memory."

"I can't imagine what that's like."

"I often wish I could watch from inside his head. You know, join him as he rebuilds his reality."

"Liz's death still hurts, but that loss was fixed in time." Jack's voice was deep and warm. "Your loss, and Jeff's, is still evolving. More like a flood than a tornado."

"That says it. Precisely. Most people don't have a clue what brain injury is like."

"I wish there were more I could do to help."

"It helps that you understand, more than you know." They talked about Kayla and Ben and the fact that Cate had lots of support. "Family, friends, and work keep me going."

"Then let's work," said Jack.

They spent an hour finalizing the journal article, discussing where to send it, and chose the *Journal of International Business Studies*, ideal for an article that explores how culture and business interact. They moved to the graduate course they would co-teach in the spring. With the PowerPoint on both computers, batting ideas back and forth, they fine-tuned the content of each slide. Jack might be the senior faculty member, but they always worked as equals, one of the reasons Cate liked him so much.

"That was a good morning's work," said Jack.

Cate chuckled. It was now midnight in Fukushima and ten in the morning in Minneapolis.

"If you're not too tired, there is something else on my mind," said Cate. "It's about Jennifer. She told me what she said to you." Across the phone lines, Cate sensed a scowl that matched hers. "She actually told you that I was busy and distracted? That she could help by co-teaching our course instead of me, that she could help with the article we just completed and add her name as coauthor?"

"She said it would be easier for you."

"The hell it would. She didn't bother to ask me."

"Jennifer's good at advancing her career. One day, if she doesn't screw up, she'll be a department chair somewhere."

"She's supposed to be my friend, not undermine me. We just collaborated on a symposium."

"Sometimes her ambition gets in her way, but for the most part, she's a good person."

"Most part isn't good enough. She knows I'm pissed, but I have to confront her more directly, Jack."

"That's fine with me. I told her I'd discuss her offers with you. If you want, let me know how the discussion goes."

"I will. Thanks again. I'll see you in a couple of months," said Cate.

"In six weeks. In the meantime, stay in touch. Text and email work, but I prefer hearing your voice. When I get back to Minneapolis, let's take a run in the Fieldhouse, or outside if the middle of March is warm enough."

* * *

After the call, Cate sat at her desk, revising her fall class, updating some slides, adding or discarding others. The popular course, *Followership, the Twin of Leadership,* taught that a huge majority of successful people in every business were followers—hardworking, confident, with excellent judgment. Few were leaders. Effective managers created an environment that freed rather than constrained follower creativity. The course, aimed at junior and senior undergraduates, which consistently had more hopeful registrants than spaces, forced students to wrestle with the concept of followership and reassess their own skills and attributes.

As she worked, Cate thought about her marriage. In the past, she and Jeff had managed to be both leaders and followers, exchanging roles, respecting competence.

When Cate finished with the revision, it was noon, but she wasn't hungry. She stood and stretched and sorted through the issues raised by Jeff's impending dress rehearsal and discharge and thought about her conversation with Jack.

It helped that work enlivened her and rarely felt like drudgery. She loved her office, her desk, and bookshelves filled with books and projects, and her wine-red chair. Framed teaching awards from graduate and undergraduate students hung on her office walls, along with family photographs, lots of them, and pictures of the narrow streets and courtyards of Aix-en-Provence from her junior year abroad and the summer in Cape Town. All the filaments of her life.

One framed photo of Jeff stood alone on the bookshelf, the image turned to face the wall in the way she had placed it a few days before Jeff's accident, imagining life without him. The memory took her breath away. She'd meant to return it to its hook but had forgotten. With a sense of urgency, she hung the picture on the wall and sat, studying it, Jeff in a field of early May daffodils at the Arboretum, his face eager and alive. They both loved daffodils, the subtle differences among varieties in the shapes and colors of cups and saucers, some with double cups or double saucers, shades from pale yellow to orange. Still in her coat, Cate gazed at the empty bottle of Saint-Emilion Grand Cru that rested on the bookshelf.

Jennifer peeked in. "Is this a good time?"

"Not really." Cate made no effort to conceal her displeasure. Jennifer's face showed surprise, then recognition, as she closed the door.

"I'm sure you talked to Jack, and I owe you a huge apology."

"Good timing. I was reviewing a draft of the Proceedings and wishing I could exclude you from authorship." Cate had decided not to permit a soft landing. "I'd like to see how you wriggle your way out of this. Or try."

"If I wanted to help you, I should have come directly to you."

"Why didn't you?"

"It came up when I was talking to Jack. At the time, it seemed like a way to help you and an opportunity for me. At least that's what I told myself."

"That's pretty lame."

"I'm not making excuses. I fucked up. I'm supposed to be your friend, and I wasn't."

"No, you weren't. Hell, you and I just ran a symposium together. We teach about values."

"What I did is on me. I'll do everything I can to rebuild your trust."

"That will take time," said Cate.

"I know. Look, I want to say one more thing," said Jennifer. "Sometimes I'm jealous about your collaboration with Jack, your friendship too—he likes you a lot—but mainly your work together, the way he respects you. I couldn't admit that to myself. If I had, I probably wouldn't have crossed that line."

"If it helps, he said you're a good person, when your ambition doesn't get in the way."

"He said that to me, too, after he scolded me."

"Well, I'm going over Rosie's draft of the Proceedings," said Cate. "I'll give it to you when I'm done."

"Then we can meet with Rosie," said Jennifer. "I know you like Mill Valley Kitchen. How about lunch, my treat? Whenever it works for you."

"Deal." Cate smiled, and Jennifer breathed a sigh of relief.

Jennifer left, leaving the door ajar. Cate watched her go. She picked up the draft of the Proceedings and worked on it until she concluded her edits and comments, then she placed it in a corner of her desk. Jennifer could wait and see them tomorrow.

Cate had decided to skip today's visit to the hospital. She'd spent a lot of time with Jeff the past weekend, and the rest of the week, starting with the dress rehearsal on Wednesday would be intense. Still, she felt a flicker of guilt. Meg's voice telling her to cut herself some slack rang in her head, and she picked up the phone.

"How about a walk?" said Meg. She suggested they meet at the Washington Avenue bridge, equidistant from the business and law schools, and hike across the river. When they reached Cate's favorite spot, Cate felt her tension ease.

"Okay," said Meg, "tell me about your Whac-A-Mole life." That brought tears of laughter to Cate's eyes. She talked about Jeff's upcoming visit, her conversation with Jack, how she had handled the conflict with Jennifer, and felt even better.

* * *

Following dinner, Cate played Chutes and Ladders with Kayla and Ben, a game they usually played as a family of four. Academic scholars argued about the significance of this game of sudden shifts in fortune: did they represent the result of good and bad deeds? Did they symbolize emotion? Or morality? Since the rolling of dice precluded choice, Jeff favored emotion. Cate favored morality. The kids ignored the argument and played the game.

Ten days had passed since Ben started Prozac. Cate had at first decided to defer medication, uneasy despite Copper's reassurance, but Bonnie's reports and Ben's distress persuaded her. When Ben landed on square 24 and climbed the ladder to square 57, he tapped the pawn twice before moving it and twice before releasing it to the new spot. To Cate's relief, the tapping lacked intensity. Since last Friday, he'd stopped complaining of morning nausea, stopped repacking his backpack, and seemed more relaxed about homework. "I'm gonna win," said Ben as he moved his pawn up the ladder.

"Not on your life," said Kayla, reaching for the dice, no longer treating Ben with the same gentleness. She moved ahead several spaces, followed by Cate's similar advance. Ben, who'd been ahead, landed on square 61, where a chute propelled him downward to square 29. He maneuvered his pawn down the chute and folded his arms across his chest.

"It wasn't a good spin, but I'm still gonna win."

"We'll see about that, little brother," said Kayla.

At bedtime, Kayla and Ben put on pajamas and brushed their teeth, preparing for bed. Cate suggested that each child pick out a book to read.

Kayla chose *My Life in Pink and Green,* about a twelve-year-old problem solver.

Ben picked *Captain Underpants and the Preposterous Plight of the Purple Potty People*. In this story, George and Harold use a time machine two days in a row, against the rules, and enter an alternative universe as Evil George and Evil Harold, where Captain Underpants, the superhero, has become evil Captain Blunderpants, with everything the opposite of the normal universe. It made Cate think. Did Ben and Kayla, as Evil Kayla and Evil Ben, feel responsible in some way for Jeff's injury? At least, in the book, the kids could adjust the time machine and return to the normal dimension.

Kids bring their own lives to fiction, thought Cate.

CHAPTER THIRTY-FOUR:

Wednesday, Hospital Day 66, February 6

Just before noon, Cate bundled Jeff into the car and headed home for the dress rehearsal. She parked in her usual spot in the garage, emerged, and waited, as Robin had suggested, to see what Jeff could do without prompts. Jeff, still in the passenger seat, looked across the empty space at the firewood stacked against the wall. He turned to look through the windshield at the Quarter Midget racers raised on two-by-fours beyond the front bumper and then at the door to the mudroom to the left of the racers.

"Let's go in," he said, but didn't move. Cate waited. Jeff pushed at the passenger door, frowned, then pulled the door handle and pushed the door open, but the seatbelt restrained him. He pulled on the shoulder strap with one hand and followed its path across his lap to the red release button. He fiddled with the button, the furrows on his brow deepening until the belt released and retracted. He pivoted, planted his feet on the garage floor, and stood. "In," he said again and moved around the car past the Quarter Midgets to the mudroom door.

Jeff climbed the two steps, turned the doorknob, and pushed. The door didn't open. He stared at the knob, tried again, repeated this sequence several times, then stood with his hand on the knob, bewildered. When he made no further attempts, Cate reached around him. "I have to unlock it with the key." She unlocked the door, turned the knob, and pushed the door open. Jeff surveyed the mudroom before he stepped over the threshold to stand inside the doorway, blocking Cate, who gently placed a hand on his back and moved him forward. She pointed to where coats hung on hooks and asked him to hang up his jacket. He touched his down jacket, then a hook, back and forth several times, seemed to make a connection, removed his coat and draped it over the hook.

"Would you like to go inside?" Cate asked, gently rotating him toward the kitchen door. As he turned, he looked to the right at the washer and dryer in the alcove and peered into the large pantry across from the laundry machines, then moved toward the closed kitchen door and stopped. Cate asked him to turn the knob and open the door. He did, although it seemed to Cate that the gears of his mind cranked and sputtered.

Once inside the kitchen, Jeff gazed at the kitchen island and its three chairs, the appliances, and the entry to the porch eating area. He walked onto the porch and sat in one of the four wicker chairs around the glass table, looking through the windows at the snow-covered landscape. His shoulders fell, and his face relaxed as he settled into the once-familiar chair.

"It's good to have you home, honey," said Cate.

Jeff inclined his head toward her, and the corners of his mouth curved upward, approximating a smile.

Cate waited, letting him get accustomed to his surroundings before she summoned Jeff's parents, who waited quietly in the family room. They appeared and embraced him. He smiled again. In the past, he would've stood and given them bear hugs.

"It's lunchtime, so you must be hungry," said Karen, offering to make one of his favorite sandwiches. He patted his stomach. Karen microwaved four veggie burgers, added avocado to each, topped two with sriracha for Cate and Jeff, and topped the others with ketchup. Jeff looked at the sandwich and licked his lips.

"Thank you," he said.

Cate pointed out familiar objects on the porch and in the landscape, reintroducing Jeff to his home, relieved that he seemed to follow her, although he showed little interest or emotion.

As they finished the meal, Dan asked, "Can you tell that we're inside the room and the trees are outside?" Jeff put his hand on the glass and peered at the trees. He turned and looked at the porch furnishings, then back at the trees. "Let me show you," said Dan. He led Jeff through the mudroom, opened the door from the mudroom to the patio, and walked onto the stoop, from where Jeff could look into the porch. Cate could see and hear them. "See, now we're outside, and the trees are outside too." He pointed at Cate and the others. "They're inside."

"That wasn't the slightest bit helpful," said Karen when they returned. "The idea is to help him feel comfortable, not stress him. If you want to do something useful, load the damn dishwasher."

With the cleanup complete, they sat in the family room and chatted, making sure to keep Jeff involved. Cate grew restless. During his Christmas visit, he'd remained on the ground floor. This time, Robin suggested that Cate take Jeff to every corner of the house to spark memories. After all, this was a dress rehearsal.

"Jeff, are you ready to see the upstairs?" asked Cate.

"Yes," he said, but he showed no enthusiasm

Cate guided him upstairs, feeling optimistic, if cautious. She and Jeff had created this home together, a place to enjoy their marriage and raise their children. Yet the tour felt like an archaeological dig.

She started with the children's rooms, which seemed safer. In Ben's room, Jeff examined Lego vehicles, transforming robots, Star Wars walkie-talkies, the K'nex set he had bought to teach Ben about the six simple machines, and Mazy the giraffe, whose long neck Jeff stroked from chin to chest. On the walls hung pictures of Ben racing Quarter Midgets, and in the closet, Jeff found Ben's orange and black racing helmets, seasoned with scrapes, the devices that protected Ben's neck from the racing bumps and crashes, and Ben's flame-resistant racing suit and gloves. "Whoosh," said Jeff, and made a racing motion with his arm.

"You've got it," said Cate.

Cate guided Jeff across the hall to Kayla's bedroom. Kayla had shoved the large dollhouse Jeff had built into a corner and filled a table with nail glitter, lip balm, and hair chalk. Sweaters, pullovers, jeans, and skirts littered her bed. Cate had to smile. Except for brimming bookshelves, Kayla's tween room looked as strange to Cate as it probably did to Jeff, who gravitated to the dollhouse, the familiar beanbag chair, the red skateboard he'd helped select, and the large stuffed tiger that still rested on the chest at the end of her bed. Cate told Jeff that Ben had been sleeping in Kayla's top bunk. Jeff touched the beds, top and bottom.

As Cate steered Jeff toward their bedroom, her apprehension increased. He stopped, poked his head into the children's bathroom, picked up one of the towels, rubbed it over his hands as if drying them, placed it back on the rack, and resumed the trek.

They'd designed their bedroom to feel peaceful. A bedspread of warm beige and silvery gray softened the white laminate bedframe. An abundance of framed family pictures sat on the low chests on the back wall. Beige and gray curtains, beige carpeting, a soft gray chair and ottoman, and a tiger maple antique chest of drawers, purchased on their honeymoon, added warmth. More family pictures adorned the antique chest. A beige and gray ballroom scene that had belonged to Cate's parents, which Jeff had never liked, hung above the fireplace. A colorful oil still life, a blue vase and richly colored flowers, one of Jeff's favorite pictures in the house, also from Cate's mother, hung above the bed.

As Jeff looked around, recognition, sadness, hope, even peace, flickered through his eyes, or at least Cate thought they did.

Jeff moved to the edge of the bed and sat in the exact spot where their locked bodies had landed the night before his accident. Cate held her breath. He shifted further onto the bed and lay on his back in his usual spot, head on the pillow, eyes open, and smiled. Cate took a deep breath, sat beside him, stroked his arm, touched his cheek, and rubbed her lips against his forehead and his cheek, feeling her tension ease. She walked around the bed and lay next to him, wrapped her arms gently around him, and squeezed. He returned the squeeze awkwardly.

It felt painful to lie there, so Cate excused herself, closed the door to the master bathroom, and sat on a small bench with her head in her hands until she regained composure. When she returned to the bedroom, Jeff was sitting up as if someone had placed him on the bed, a lifelike figure that didn't belong.

Cate took his arm and finished the tour. She showed him their bathroom, their walk-in closet and descended past the first floor to the finished part of the basement, where the children had a play space and where Kayla and Cate practiced gymnastics. She showed him the unfinished part, shelves he had erected to store things, including the Quarter Midget tires. They returned to the first floor, and Cate deposited him in the family room with his parents. She considered bringing him down the hall, past the mudroom and extra bathroom, to the mother-in-law space that served as her office, her sanctuary, but decided against it.

They were sitting in the family room, Cate, Jeff, and his parents, when Kayla and Ben burst into the house and greeted their dad. The children were all over him, touching him, hugging him, curling up on either side of him on the couch, telling him how happy they were to see him. Jeff responded with more animation than Cate had seen. The children sat almost in his lap.

"I'm glad you're staying overnight, Daddy, but why do you have to go back to the hospital?" asked Ben. Kayla reminded her brother that Dad would have one more night in the hospital and come home for good on Friday.

As Cate watched the interaction, she understood better the reason for the dress rehearsal. Not only would it help Jeff and make certain that no adjustments were needed before discharge, but it would also smooth Jeff's reentry into all their lives.

They sat in the family room, just being together, until dinnertime, when Dan picked up Chinese takeout.

Afterward, Ben wanted to play Trivial Pursuit, but Kayla said it wasn't a good game for Dad, so they set up Monopoly on the dining room table. Ben partnered with his dad and played against Kayla and Cate as the grandparents kibitzed. Bedtime arrived, and Cate, perched on the lower bunk with Jeff beside her, read to the children. When she tucked them into bed, Jeff imitated her by putting his hands under the mattress. Cate thanked him for helping.

"Hey," said Kayla, sitting up. "We forgot to show Dad the snow family."

"And the spirit bear," said Ben.

"It's dark outside. They'll still be there in the morning," said Cate. It took the children a few minutes to quiet down again as Cate rubbed Kayla's shoulders, and Dan imitated her by rubbing Ben's. When the kids were asleep, or close, Cate and Jeff returned to the family room and sat together opposite Jeff's parents. Jeff seemed to settle comfortably into the couch.

"Honey, when you come home for good the day after tomorrow, Copper's going to visit for a week. That will make it easier for all of us."

"We'll visit too, son, every day this weekend," said Dan.

"On Monday, I have to work," said Karen, "but we'll drive up from Northfield as often as we can." She looked at Cate and Jeff holding hands. "Dan, maybe we should leave these two lovebirds alone for a while." Jeff's parents hugged Cate and Jeff and left for the guest room.

Cate sat with Jeff, watching an old episode of *Mash*. Although he seemed to laugh at times, she could not tell how much he followed the plot or remembered the characters, but Cate didn't want to make the evening an interrogation.

At ten, once again she led Jeff upstairs, where he undressed and put on the pajamas she had placed on the bed. In the bathroom, he brushed his teeth and used the toilet, then crawled under the bedcovers and lay on his back with open eyes. Cate did her own preparations for bed and hesitated, unsure if she wanted to climb into bed or go downstairs to read. She decided on bed and lay facing him, her arm extended to touch his face the way he liked. Before the accident, this might have become foreplay. At last, Jeff's eyes closed. After looking at his sleeping form for several minutes, Cate shut her eyes and fell into a dream-filled sleep.

When she awakened, well before the alarm, Jeff was gone. Cate checked the bathroom and the children's bedrooms and, to her astonishment, found him in pajamas on the porch, eating a bowl of Cheerios, a carton of milk and a container of blueberries next to the bowl. From what Cate knew about TBI, sometimes a window opened, a memory surfaced, a behavior surprised, but it might not represent the level of function she could consistently expect. "Nice, you figured out breakfast." Cate felt proud, the kind of pride she might feel for Kayla and Ben when they accomplished a new task.

"Keurig." She followed his gaze. The lid of the Keurig was open, a ruptured K-cup crushed into it upside down, no coffee mug below. Cate had to clear the grounds from the ruptured K-cup and rinse the mechanism before guiding him through the brewing steps. The coffee smelled good and Cate, with a gulp, remembered how much Jeff used to love the smell of morning coffee. She added milk to match the rich tan color he preferred. "Enjoy the coffee and breakfast, honey. I'll get the children going."

She returned shortly, dressed, with the children in tow. "Mommy told us you made breakfast for yourself, Daddy!" said Ben. Jeff turned to him with a half-smile.

"Jeff, say good morning to Ben and Kayla."

"Good morning," he said. Kayla, ever alert, added five more bowls to the table as Karen and Dan appeared. They ate and talked, making sure to include Jeff.

"Dad, put on your coat and come with us to see the snow family and the spirit bear," said Kayla.

"Yeah, we can visit them until the bus comes," said Ben. All four adults donned coats and walked outside to stand with the snow sculpture.

"We're gonna miss seeing you tonight," said Kayla, "but tomorrow, you're coming home."

"Have a good last night in the hospital, Daddy," said Ben. The kids waved to their dad from the windows of the bus.

CHAPTER THIRTY-FIVE:

Friday, Discharge/Hospital Day 68, February 8

Kayla and Ben, who'd skipped school, waited with their dad and an unfamiliar nurse in the morning cold while Cate fetched the car from the ramp. By the time she pulled up, Jane had joined the group and greeted Cate with a smile. "We couldn't let Jeff leave without a warm sendoff," she said and handed him a picture of his entire Knapp treatment team gathered around him, smiling broadly. "Every one of us will miss you and your family." She hugged Jeff and Cate and the children. "You'll be in good hands at Sister Kenny, Jeff, but remember to stay in touch. We'd love to hear about your progress." Jeff nodded and smiled, but the smile held no anticipation. Cate, excited and apprehensive, shed tears for both of them.

"Everyone has been great," she said. "We can never thank you enough. We'll miss you, and of course we'll keep you in the loop."

"Before you go, one last picture." The unfamiliar nurse snapped a photo of Jeff with his family and Jane. Then Cate bundled Jeff into the passenger seat, stowed the suitcase and a plastic bag of extra gear in the trunk, belted Jeff into the car, made sure the children wore seatbelts, and drove off.

"You're coming home, Daddy!" said Ben, who put his arms around his dad's neck. Kayla, seated behind Cate, patted his shoulder.

"Yes, I am." Jeff clasped his hands around an imaginary steering wheel.

Cate negotiated the city streets, heading for the highway, trying to imagine what Jeff might be like in the next few weeks and months. In the rearview mirror, Kayla and Ben chatted happily, and Jeff, not quite inert, sat beside her.

In the garage, they exited the car and walked through the mudroom to the kitchen, Cate carrying the suitcase, Kayla the plastic bag, Ben holding his dad's hand. Karen and Dan greeted Jeff with hugs. Dan carried the luggage upstairs as Karen guided Jeff to the family room. Everyone relaxed for an hour or so, talking quietly, letting Jeff acclimate. It felt easier than the dress rehearsal.

They moved to the porch for lunch and had barely begun to eat when Copper arrived by cab from the airport. She insisted that everyone keep eating.

"Hello, Copper; nice to see you," said Jeff, his voice too loud, yet his language and responsiveness raised Cate's eyebrows.

"Hi, Jeff. It's nice to see you at home."

"Home?" Jeff studied his surroundings.

"I'm glad you're home, Daddy," said Ben, leaning his head against his dad. Kayla, on his other side, rested a hand on his arm. Jeff put down his sandwich and reached for his children.

When they finished lunch, Jeff carried his dish to the sink, rinsed it, and placed it in the dishwasher. Cate watched, wishing his behavior were more consistent, predictable. Dan did the rest of the cleanup and joined everyone in the family room, except for Copper, who went upstairs to unpack.

"Dad, do you understand you're not going back to the hospital? You're home for good?" asked Kayla. He surveyed the furniture, décor, the fire Ben had helped him start, and the large windows that overlooked the front yard. He did a second survey focused on people. Slowly a look of contentment spread across his face.

"I'm staying home," he said. "No more hospital." The children curled against him.

"Dad, put your arms around us like you used to," said Kayla. Jeff rested his arms on their shoulders so quietly that he almost disappeared into the chair. Cate thought about turning on the TV, but Jeff seemed content, and everyone else was chatting amiably. As the flames grew smaller and the embers glowed with less intensity, Ben followed his dad's eyes to the fading embers.

"I want that fire to burn bright red for you, Daddy," said Ben. "Let's put some *big* logs on." Ben took his dad's hand, and they selected from the wood basket a birch log with peeling bark and a piece of sturdy oak, thick and heavy, added it, and returned to the couch, watching the flames.

Outside, a snowfall had begun. "Daddy, now that you're home for good, we have to go see the spirit bear and the snow family before the snow covers them up," said Ben.

"They'll still be there, under the snow," said Dan.

"And we can use the new snow if they need repair," said Karen.

"But Ben's right. We have to go outside. We should visit them now," said Kayla.

Everyone put on coats and hats and followed Ben and Kayla into the falling snow to visit the six snow people and the spirit bear. Jeff walked first to the humans, touching each figure in turn, then rested a gloved hand on the spirit bear.

"Let's add Aunt Copper to the snow family," said Kayla.

"Yeah," said Ben.

"I'd be honored," said Copper. The kids rolled two snowballs and stacked them with Cate and Dan's help. Karen molded two rods of snow, partly supported by the shoulder of the new figure, connected the rods, and shaped them.

"I know what that is," said Kayla. "It's a trombone."

"You guessed right," said Karen. She re-draped one of the long scarves to bring Copper into the snow family. Kayla ran into the house and returned with a green wool cap and two buttons for snow Copper's eyes.

At Copper's suggestion, they formed a hugging circle, a group hug, in front of the spirit bear as fresh snow made all the figures white and fresh. Dan took out his phone. "Hey, I have a selfie stick," said Kayla, and she raced into the house once more. She had to show Dan how to use it, and it took several tries to get all the figures in the picture, but Dan succeeded. He said he'd email it to everyone and have a copy printed for the gallery in the back hall.

Everyone returned to the family room and sat talking. Ben's eyes searched the room. "Where's your trombone, Aunt Copper?" said Ben.

"I didn't bring it this time. But I brought some very special trombone CDs." She produced three gift-wrapped packages and gave the bigger one to Jeff. He tore open the wrapping and found a three-CD set, Tommy Dorsey and His Orchestra.

"Cate, will you play the first song on disc two?" said Cate. "It's one of Dorsey's trademark songs, and it's perfect for Jeff." They listened to Tommy's trombone and his big band, gentle and evocative, play *I'm Getting Sentimental Over You.* After a few more songs on that disc, Copper held out two CDs. "Whatever you find when you unwrap yours, they're both good. Ben found Chris Brubeck, and Kayla found Delfeayo Marsalis. "Now you have CDs of my three favorite trombonists."

"*You're* my favorite," said Kayla. "Do you have a CD?"

"Not yet, but we're talking to a recording studio."

"Can I have one when it's done?" said Ben.

"You bet. You guys can have the first one."

For the rest of the afternoon, they listened to trombone music and talked. From time to time, they glanced out the window at the snow sculpture, blurred by falling snow, standing tall.

* * *

It was an easy supper for Jeff's first night home—Muenster cheeseburgers made by Copper in a skillet. Before the accident, Jeff would have shoveled a path through patio snow and grilled them.

After dinner, they retired to the living room for a concert the kids had prepared to celebrate Jeff's homecoming. Two weeks ago, with

Cate's gentle urging, the kids had resumed music practice. Kayla and Ben had played since they were five, each starting Suzuki violin lessons with Miss Jennifer in nearby Minnetonka, modified Suzuki because they learned to read music. At seven, Kayla switched to piano and began lessons at MacPhail Center for Music in downtown Minneapolis, a longer schlep, another kid activity that Cate would have to keep going, along with Kayla's piano quartet at MacPhail. Ben continued violin lessons with Miss Jennifer. Jeff would joke that everyone, including Cate, played an instrument and all he played was the radio.

Jeff always worried that the kids were overscheduled with music, gymnastics, Quarter Midget racing, and dancing, but they were no busier than their friends and enjoyed what they did, so he and Cate had shared the burden. Now all of this would fall to Cate, with Mandy's help.

Ben, surveying his attentive audience, especially his dad, put his fingers in third position on the fingerboard and soloed Dvořák's *Humoresque* with self-conscious vibrato, followed by a gavotte with Kayla's piano accompaniment, all from Suzuki music books. Jeff smiled and noiselessly put his hands together.

"Hey Jeff, did you forget how to clap?" Cate showed him, and the kids smiled at his audible applause. Then Kayla played a Mozart piano sonata and Mendelssohn's *Venetian Gondola Song* from the Suzuki book. Jeff closed his eyes and swayed slightly to the music. As the others applauded, Jeff's claps grew louder and more defined.

"Play with us, Mom," said Kayla. Cate withdrew her violin from its case atop the piano and played a Suzuki duet with Ben, accompanied by Kayla on piano. The kids played a few more pieces, solo or violin and piano duets. By the time the recital concluded, Jeff was clapping easily.

At the kids' bedtime, everyone climbed the stairs, Kayla and Ben gripping their dad's hands. Jeff sat on the edge of Kayla's bed with Cate next to him, Ben beside Kayla, the others listening. When the story was over, both kids hugged their parents.

"You're home, Daddy," said Ben, his eyes shining. Jeff puckered his lips and kissed his children on their foreheads. Everyone said goodnight.

Jeff's parents left for Northfield, and Copper retreated to the guestroom, allowing Cate and Jeff time alone. Cate had planned to return to the family room, but Jeff headed for the bedroom. He looked around and sat easily on the bed, more naturally than two days earlier. With minimal prompting, he showered and changed into the pajamas that Cate had set out for him. Cate noticed that he was thinner, his body less muscular, the huge scar on his left shoulder more prominent. Cate loved that scar, the only flaw on his body. He lay down without turning out the light, without saying goodnight to Cate, eyes open.

"You don't look like you're ready for sleep. Want to sit up and watch TV?" Cate arranged the pillows so they could sit comfortably and turned on the set. She'd heard about a new Netflix series, and they watched the first episode of *House of Cards*. She liked it. Jeff watched without interest.

When the episode was over, Jeff adjusted his pillow and lay down, staring at the ceiling. Cate got out of bed, brushed her teeth, and slipped into a nightgown. Perched on his side of the bed, she kissed his forehead and cheeks and felt a familiar stirring, muted by his lack of interest. She thought they should at least hug, which she would have to initiate, but felt little urge, more obligation than desire. She shut off his bedside light, returned to her side of the bed, placed her hands against his cheeks, and kissed him. He returned the kiss but did not touch her. She felt unsure whether to pursue him or wait, wondering what was best for him. *Caregiver, a good caregiver.* That's what one of the nurses had called her.

Where there should be mutual stirrings, there was only desolation. She told herself this was a new beginning, that she had to be patient, to wait for things to improve. He was home, and that was good.

She faced the wall, dispirited and filled with grief, sobbing quietly until her emotions settled. When she looked again at Jeff, he was asleep. A familiar object in a familiar place.

Cate read, trying to quiet her mind. When she felt tired, finally, she kissed Jeff's cheek. "Welcome home," she whispered, hoping, and fell into a troubled sleep.

CHAPTER THIRTY-SIX:

Home, Monday, February 11

On Monday morning, Cate roused Jeff so he could have breakfast with the children, just the four of them. It was Copper's idea; she waited in the guestroom. Jeff sat quietly at the table, but to Cate, he seemed more present, more aware of the kids and their conversation. As the children donned coats, Jeff poured milk into their empty cereal bowls.

"Thanks, Daddy," said Ben, "but I'm done."

Kayla ate one spoonful of the extra milk and hugged her dad goodbye.

Ben didn't get sick that morning, loaded his backpack without problems, and worried only a little about homework, including the extra work his teacher emailed to Cate because Ben had missed school on Friday. Kayla, on her own, had arranged to make up Friday's work.

When the kids were gone, Cate poured Jeff more coffee. "It's fun to see you in the morning, honey," said Cate.

"It is fun," said Jeff, with half a grin.

"You too, Copper," said Cate as she appeared and made herself breakfast. "I appreciate how hard it is to get away for a week when you have a four-year-old."

"Will was glad to have father-daughter time. He and Sophia will be fine."

"Aren't Will's parents available?"

"They offered, but it seemed like more fun without them. Sophia does have nursery school during the week, so he'll get some work done. Anyway, I'm here. It's sister time, and your kids love me."

Cate laughed. "Haven't heard 'sister time' since we were kids."

"Jeffie loves me too. Don't you, brother-in-law?" Jeff's face bobbed several times.

"You make everything cheerful," said Cate. "That's why we love you."

"You can go to work and know everything here is good."

"Good," said Jeff.

"I do have to work, but Copper will keep you laughing." Cate retrieved her coat from the mudroom, returned to the eating area, and kissed Jeff. "Hard to believe, but you're home, and I'm going to work." Jeff's brow furrowed. "Honey, it's another milestone."

"He'll understand in time, won't you, Jeffie?" said Copper.

"Okay, you two have a fun day," said Cate.

Copper turned to Jeff. "What's your pleasure? Trombone music or Mozart?"

"I like Copper's trombone," he said as Cate walked into the mudroom and out the door with a light step.

She drove, relishing the sunny day and the fresh snow that covered the ground but had melted from the streets.

CHAPTER THIRTY-SEVEN:

Wednesday, February 13

Cate steeled herself for an arduous day. This morning, she and Jeff would meet with Jeff's new occupational therapist to work on cognition. In the rehab world, cognition meant more than knowledge and understanding. It meant marshaling specific skills to address everything from kitchen chores to planning one's day. Cognitive OT was the approach that would bring Jeff fully back from his TBI or help him adjust to permanent disability.

Lori Bradshaw, the Cognitive OT therapist, greeted them and asked Jeff if he remembered what they planned to work on today.

"No," he said, uninterested.

"Honey, you have to care," said Cate. "You have to try."

"Okay," said Jeff in a dreary voice.

"This is for you, honey. I know you have good days and bad. Please, if you can, make this a good one."

"Today, looks like we should start with the basics," said Lori, positioning herself directly in front of Jeff, touching his shoulder. "Why do you come to see me?" Jeff didn't answer, but he narrowed his eyes, concentrating. "When I tell you that you had a brain injury, does that sound familiar?" Jeff nodded, leaning forward. Cate relaxed a bit; Lori knew how to reach him.

"Good. You know that you have a TBI. Today, we're going to work on understanding how that TBI affects you. Are you with me?"

"Yes," said Jeff. His voice had acquired color, and his face showed animation.

"We're going to start with *awareness.*" Lori explained that Jeff functioned at the most basic level of awareness, *intellectual awareness.* He knew he had a brain injury. The next step was to extend that level of awareness, so Jeff knew how his brain injury affected him. Lori had given him a notebook, called *Jeff's Logbook,* to carry everywhere, which he clutched. "You remembered the logbook," she said. "That's also intellectual awareness, knowing you need the logbook." She helped Jeff write in the logbook, "I have a brain injury," and below that, "I have to write things down to remember them."

"You're going to use the logbook to write down assignments to do at home," she glanced at Cate, "and Cate's going to help you work on them. She's going to be my co-therapist. Here's the first assignment." Following Lori's instructions, Jeff wrote, *Pick something I do well, like showering, and break it into steps.* "Here's what I mean," said Lori. "Getting the towel ready, letting the shower run to get warm, shampoo and rinse, soap your body and rinse, dry." Once Jeff practiced and could do that easily, Lori wanted him to use the same approach for something more difficult, like picking out clothes that match or making a salad. He wrote, *Choose something hard (Cate can help), and do the same thing.* Then, *Practice twice a day for fifteen minutes.* "Do you understand?"

He looked at what he had written, at Cate, and nodded.

Cate asked about the other levels of awareness. After intellectual awareness, Lori explained, the next stage was *emergent awareness,* the ability to recognize a problem as it occurs. For example, as Jeff loads the dishwasher, he might notice that he gets flustered. Or he might note irritability when the whole family gets together.

The highest level of awareness, *anticipatory awareness,* involves the ability to know in advance that a problem would occur and plan a strategy to cope with it. If Jeff knows that he gets tired every evening, he might plan an afternoon nap. "That's when Cognitive OT really gets going," said Lori. "Eventually, with luck, we'll use it to plan a simple task at work, then more complex tasks. But that's far down the road."

Cate gulped.

"I know we have a long way to go. Did you understand the homework part?"

"Yes. I'm beginning to see how this works," said Cate.

"Good, because a lot depends on homework. In Cognitive OT, we leverage what Jeff can do to build new skills. It's not just that his brain is healing; what we do helps his brain rewire."

They agreed to meet weekly, with Cate attending part of each session. Lori would meet with Jeff three times a week. As Jeff improved over the next several months, they'd meet less frequently. He'd eventually learn to use the logbook to communicate homework assignments, and Cate could come less often.

The session ended, and Cate checked her watch. She hadn't taken Jeff to see *Wellspring* in the hospital courtyard. There was time before Jeff's next appointment, and Cate thought they both needed inspiration. They walked outside and discovered it was warm enough to linger. Cate pointed to the bronze family, arms reaching upward. "A wellspring is where things begin. A source. Does that make sense to you?" Jeff shook his head. "Then think of it this way; it's about hope."

"Hope," said Jeff. His eyes followed the arms into the sky.

"Your mom knows the sculptor who made this. She did a workshop with him. Some of his work will be in the new sculpture garden at the Arboretum."

"Let's see it at the Arboretum?"

"That's right. Sometimes you surprise me."

"Thank you."

Cate checked her watch. "It's time for us to meet with the neuropsychologist."

"He did my testing."

"That's right."

They walked to the office of Dr. Bill Bartlett, whom Cate had not yet met, and he greeted them warmly. Although his office felt inviting, and his manner was friendly, Cate imagined him in judicial robes: when it came to understanding Jeff's behavior and capacities, neuropsychology was the Supreme Court.

Behind his desk hung a framed origami picture labeled *One Thousand Cranes,* and colorful origami animals, flowers, and folded pyramids crammed shelves in front of books and journals and littered his desk. The office resembled an origami palace, and Cate could not resist a smile.

"Do you like origami?" he asked.

"I do, but not as much as you."

"Most of the folded ones on the bookshelves were made by disabled patients. My wife helped my kids make some of the complex ones, like the crimson lily and the elephant. It's a hobby my family loves, and I introduce to disabled artists."

"How about the picture?"

"A patient made that. Japanese myth says that gods will grant a wish to anyone who folds one thousand cranes. In rehab, it's the work, the perseverance that fulfills the wish."

Cate looked at Jeff.

Dr. Bartlett brushed a lock of hair from his forehead. "So, to business. Jeff, is it okay if I talk to Cate about you?"

"Yes."

"I assume you've heard the trope, 'marathon-not-a-sprint?'"

"I run marathons. They have a set path and a clear endpoint."

"I can't disagree, but stay with the metaphor. As Jeff runs the TBI marathon, testing will help illuminate his path and, eventually, it will clarify the endpoint."

"Okay. I get that," said Cate.

"I see from the record that you're a psychologist."

"Organizational psychology. I teach leadership in the business school at the U and do a little executive coaching. It's not like seeing patients in an office."

"May I assume you're familiar with basic stuff like Wechsler IQ testing and MMPI personality assessment?"

"Of course."

"Any neuropsychology along the way?"

"One course in graduate school. Brain injury is out of my league."

"Tell me what you remember about neuropsych."

"It's a way to evaluate the kinds of skills an executive uses at work: attention, memory, judgment, the ability to manipulate ideas and make decisions, plan for the future, use language to communicate ideas."

"That's a good description. I'd add visual-spatial skills, important for basic things like navigating around a house or driving through a neighborhood, and for you, Jeff, telling one end of a cow from the other."

Cate smiled.

"I'd also add social-emotional functioning," he continued, "which includes drive and initiative, the way Jeff communicates with and interacts with others, his emotional tone or lack of it."

"Jeff used to excel in all those areas," said Cate, with an audible sigh, taking Jeff's hand.

"He's a bright and creative guy, and that helps." He smiled at Jeff. "Yet it's not surprising that he has problems in some of these areas, including motivation and social communication. On the positive side, his language function, as you know, is quite good. His visual-spatial skills are intact and have never shown impairment."

Cate leaned forward, a protective hand on Jeff's arm.

"In general, the neuropsych tests confirm what we might expect—no surprises, but it does help to define where we are on the path and where Jeff's heading," said Dr. Bartlett. "It's useful information for Lori as she extends Jeff's cognitive abilities."

Cate nodded, hoping for some reaction from Jeff.

"All of these skills interact," he said. "For example, even though language skills are good, Jeff could not read a novel because of problems with attention and memory."

"What about insight and awareness?"

"Insight, awareness, judgment, warmth, and humor all require intact frontal lobes and intact connections of frontal lobes with other parts of the brain. We find deficits in all these areas on testing, as expected with diffuse axonal injury. Remember, it's early in the marathon."

"How do you measure personality?"

"Personality, which the MMPI describes, tracks more or less with higher cognitive functions. But it's important to remember that personality changes might persist, independent of improved cognition."

Cate felt lost, as if a bridge necessary to reach home had partially washed away. She had many questions but could articulate none.

"While the MMPI and neuropsych tests provide useful information about personality," Dr. Bartlett continued, "how Jeff behaves in the real world, his drive and his interactions with others, is the ultimate measure."

"His actual behavior?"

"That's the acid test, but every bit of information is important in understanding Jeff and guiding treatment."

"When do you put it all together?"

"We keep making determinations as long as additional recovery is possible. As you know, that's roughly two years from injury."

"Unless he recovers completely before that?"

"Yes. And I wish that were likely."

"Any other endpoint?"

"For effort, choose your yardstick." Dr. Bartlett smiled. "One thousand cranes or 26.2 miles."

Cate sighed.

"The closer we get, the sharper the focus, the brighter the illumination. Jeff, as time passes, you and Cate will have a lot better idea of where and how this ends. You'll have lots of time to adjust and lots of help and support. In the meantime, call anytime you have concerns."

Neither of them had questions, and they left, thanking Dr. Bartlett.

On the way home, Cate stopped. While Jeff waited in the car outside a bakery, Cate picked up a heart-shaped cake.

Tomorrow was Valentine's Day.

CHAPTER THIRTY-EIGHT:

Friday, February 15

Cate's alarm blared at 6:45. She dressed, awakened Jeff, and they descended to the kitchen, where the kids were scarfing down flapjacks and laughing with Copper. Last night, Copper had mixed the flapjack ingredients and early this morning, tossed them in the oven, giving them time to cool. The flapjacks, thick and square and made with rolled oats, dried dates, butter, and sugar, were a parting gift. "Something special for special kids," said Copper.

"I wish you didn't have to go," said Ben.

"Before I leave tonight, let's call Sophia. I promised her she could say hi to everyone once more before I go."

"I'll bet she misses you," said Ben.

"Aunt Copper says we might all go to Cape Cod this summer and rent a house, like we did last summer," said Kayla.

"Daddy likes it there," said Ben.

Jeff cocked his head and grinned.

"I have a gift for Sophia from Ben and me," said Kayla, handing Copper a copy of *Harold and the Purple Crayon.* She'd stuffed the gift bag with tissue paper and taped a purple crayon inside.

"Mommy showed us how to wrap it," said Ben. "Daddy helped too."

"A gift for Sophia," said Jeff.

"It's a perfect gift because Sophia is learning to read," said Copper.

"Aunt Copper, can all four-year-olds read?" asked Ben.

"Only smart ones like you and Kayla."

It was time to leave for school, but one pan of flapjacks remained. "That's so you remember me when you have breakfast tomorrow," said Copper

"We'll remember," said Kayla.

"On your way," said Cate. "Aunt Copper isn't leaving until tonight, so you'll see her again before she leaves." Kayla and Ben hugged Copper and left.

* * *

In the Sister Kenny elevator, Cate pressed the button for the second floor, turned to face Jeff, and searched his eyes. "Do you remember why we're here today?"

"No."

"To see Dr. Hunter, the psychologist. You've met him and so have I, when we first came to Sister Kenny. You've improved enough to benefit from talking. Maybe it will help you, and us." Cate willed herself to smile. The lower part of Jeff's face, but not his eyes, responded.

"I wish I knew how to read you," she said as the elevator doors opened, and they took a seat in the reception area.

Shortly, Dr. Hunter appeared. "It's good to see you again," he said. He ushered them to his office, and they sat in front of a grainy plastic desk on which rested a vase of daffodils. It seemed like everyone in Minnesota bought daffodils in February. Behind him hung a streetscape with exuberant colors, buildings that thrust triumphantly into an azure sky. Cate knew it was another painting by a disabled artist.

"That picture is nice," said Jeff.

"It's the first-prize watercolor from the last year's art show," said Dr. Hunter.

"It's stunning. What kind of injury did that person have?" asked Cate.

"Quadriplegia, with limited use of his arms."

"Not a brain injury?"

"No."

Cate nodded. Her mouth felt dry. She moved her tongue around her mouth, sucking, trying to generate saliva. Dr. Hunter offered her a bottled water.

"Thanks," said Cate, taking Jeff's hand, studying his expressionless face. Tearing up, she looked back at Dr. Hunter. "It's hard to see Jeff like this. Before the accident, he was full of life."

"Brain injury has special challenges. My role is to help both of you adapt to an evolving reality, individually and as a couple. How are you both doing?" Neither replied. "How about you, Cate?"

"Anxious, exhausted, and very sad."

"I've never seen a spouse who wasn't. Most see me or seek their own professional help."

"Talking to friends has worked so far."

"It's hard to acknowledge what has changed, that your spouse isn't the same."

"Besides work, which I love, I get together with friends, one in particular whom I've known since college. I have strong family support. Overall, I'm managing."

"That's good. Jeff, how about you?"

"It's okay," said Jeff, without emotion.

"You're okay?"

"Yes."

"Do you want to comment, Cate?"

"Honey, you react to me and the kids, but you don't initiate things, and you don't show much emotion. I wouldn't call that okay, but I know you're doing the best you can."

"That describes very well what we often see following a brain injury. We call it lack of drive, apathy, as I think you know. Usually, there are emotions that exist alongside apathy. Jeff, you might feel bored, frustrated, tired, or angry. I can help you recognize that part of your experience. As you gain more insight, you'll have more feelings. I'd suggest that we meet once a week to talk about what's happening."

"It's very hard to see triumphant buildings in our future," said Cate, gesturing at the painting behind Dr. Hunter, "as much as I'd love to be optimistic. It all looks gray."

"Now that Jeff's home, you've moved from survival mode to long-term adjustment. From acute anxiety to chronic apprehension. Things are still settling, so there's a lot of uncertainty, and that can be harder than tragedy."

Jeff shifted in his chair, restless. His face grew tight.

"See? That's not apathy. Tell me what you're feeling."

"Nervous."

"That's an unpleasant feeling, but it reflects insight. What are you nervous about?"

"I don't know."

"I think I know. We're talking about Cate's expectations and fears, her sadness. You're responding to her emotion." Jeff looked at Cate and sat rigidly in the chair.

"It's okay, honey." Cate touched his arm. He leaned back, and his face softened.

"That's a good example of how you affect each other. It's worth recognizing, and part of what we can work on together."

"Maybe it's a good idea to meet as a couple," said Cate.

"I was hoping you'd say that. Once a month, we can make our weekly visit a couple's session. Would that work?"

They both agreed.

"Then we have a plan. You might think of brain injury as an earthquake that destroys the usual landmarks, so it's hard to find your way. I can help you with that. I can't live in your shoes, but I can travel that path with you."

* * *

Karen and Dan arrived for an early dinner, which allowed time for a Skype visit with Sophia before her bedtime and before Copper left for the airport. They gathered around the computer. "Look at me, Mom," said Sophia. "I'm wearing an apron. Dad bought it for me because I wanted to be like you."

"You look cute, sweetie," said Copper.

"Dad says you're coming home tonight, but you're still there."

"I'm going to the airport very soon."

"Hi, Sophia." Ben waved at the computer, and Sophia waved back.

"Mom told us we might all go to Cape Cod this summer," said Ben. "Then we can see you without the computer."

Kayla reached for her dad and pulled him in front of the screen. "Look, Sophia. My dad's home." Kayla took his hand and waved it. When she released it, he continued waving.

"Your home, with my mom?" asked Sophia.

"Yes, sweetie. We loved having your mom here. Is it okay if we send her back to you?" said Cate.

"Yes! I want my mom."

"I'll see you very soon, my love," said Copper.

They talked for several more minutes. Kayla and Ben said hi to Uncle Bill, who told Jeff he was looking good and sent hugs. Then Copper picked up her suitcase and Sophia's gift bag and left with Karen and Dan, who'd bring her to the airport.

For Cate, it was the end of a long week and a very long day. She sat with Jeff and with Kayla and Ben in the family room, watching TV, thinking about the future.

In twelve days, Kayla would turn eleven. Cate still had to plan the party.

CHAPTER THIRTY-NINE:

Saturday, end of March

Cate wanted to run. When Meg arrived, she was ready to go. On the fourth weekend in March, the outside temperature had reached fifty degrees. Since Minnesota blizzards sometimes occur in April, they wanted to take advantage of the beautiful day. Only traces of snow survived, the sun glistened, and running would keep them warm with light jackets. Scott would take a walk with Jeff while the kids played.

Spring break at the university had ended two days ago, and already Cate felt tired, a pleasant kind of tired because her life felt more or less on track, the best track possible, all things considered. She had established Jeff's daily and weekly routine, and the kids had adapted well. Ben was doing better at school, less anxious, and Kayla was thriving. In the past two days, Cate had sent the symposium Proceedings to the publisher, started to teach her spring undergraduate class, met with all her graduate students, had a quick run with Jack in the Fieldhouse, and submitted the paper she and Jack coauthored after a few minor edits.

She was glad for today's respite since this year, the kids didn't have spring break until the following week, and the grandparents had obligations for part of that week, so she'd be stretched thin. Between Cate and Meg, with help from Mandy, she had the week covered with playdates and other plans. Although Kayla and Evie were now eleven and could watch their younger brothers without supervision, the moms wanted to fill vacation week with fun, not responsibility.

Meg and Cate piled into Meg's car, drove the mile to their favorite Caribou coffee shop, parked, crossed the street to the hiking trail behind the grocery store, and jogged west for two miles at a pace slow enough to converse, then raced for a mile. They returned at a brisk pace, crossed the street, and collapsed with agreeable fatigue into coffee shop chairs and sat around a wood table, sipping decaf lattes, without talking. It was Cate who broke the silence. "That felt surprisingly good. Except for once or twice with you, and basement gymnastics with the kids, I haven't gotten much exercise recently."

"You didn't count your run with Jack."

"Guess not. That was Wednesday."

"When did he get back?"

"To the States, ten days ago. He spent the first few days with his sons and families on the East Coast and got here Tuesday."

"Then you didn't waste much time."

"Cut it out. He's a good guy, and it was nice to see him."

"When are you getting together again?"

"Haven't planned it, but I'm sure we'll run into each other. We talked about a run along the river near his place."

"You like him a lot, so be careful."

"Can't you think of anything else? It's under control."

"That's good to hear."

"Thank you."

"Actually, before Jack came up, I was thinking about Jeff and the accident and how well, overall, all of you have adapted. It's been a crazy few months."

"Close to four. There are still days I don't want to get out of bed, and days I don't want to stay there because some guy who looks like Jeff—but isn't Jeff—is there."

"Have you gone to that TBI support group you told me about?"

"Once last week, during the break. Families of vets and accident victims, some athletes. Now I understand all the newspaper articles about people who've lost part of themselves and aren't the same."

"A lot of these people are younger than Jeff, aren't they?

"Most of the vets are, and many of the accident victims. Football players are older; they have more headaches, irritability, mood swings, and bigger risk of suicide."

"Are you worried about suicide?"

"Not with Jeff. I'm worried about apathy." Cate swallowed. She looked away and teared. "I never told you the details of the fight we had the night before the accident. At the time, I was furious that Jeff had the gall to be angry too, but now I'd give anything to feel that anger. God, it was a good and healthy fight."

"What did happen that night?"

"He approached me in heat. Instead of responding like I usually do, I exploded. I told him that sex was the only way we interacted, that I didn't want a marriage based on fucking."

"How did he respond?"

"At first, he was surprised. When my anger grew, instead of abating, he blew up and blamed me for the distance. He said he couldn't talk to me because I run from confrontation, that I'm making the kids as scared as me. We were close enough to spit, and it got hotter and hotter."

"Were you worried? Anger and sex are a dangerous combination."

"No. He was never abusive. We were in each other's faces, but we kept our voices low so that the kids wouldn't hear, and I was the one who lost it. I went after him, pushed him onto the bed, yanked off his underpants, brought him to the edge, and kept him there for a while until I was satisfied. It was hot and passionate for both of us."

"Wow."

"I've thought about that night a lot. The funny thing is, in retrospect, Jeff described me accurately, and that's not the person I want to be. We both used anger and arousal to bridge the distance, yet there was something honest about it. By the next morning, we felt a lot less angry. Even close. We were going to talk that evening."

"And then the accident."

"Yes. We fought about distance, and now that's all there is; he's here, but he's not here. I'm terrified about what I've lost, what the kids have lost. Most of all, I'm terrified because Jeff isn't."

"God, Cate." Meg had tears in her eyes. "Wish I knew what to say."

"You listen, and that's what I need."

"I was thinking that the run felt good for both of us. I should have let you enjoy the day."

"Don't apologize. It's always there below the surface." Cate stretched. "Would you mind another run, a half mile or so?"

"I think both of us could use that." They crossed the street to the path. When they'd run a quarter mile and were ready to return, they decided to double it. They finished the run with a strong kick.

CHAPTER FORTY:

April

Cate's neck was in knots, and her stomach reminded her that she'd skipped breakfast. At one o'clock, tired and discouraged, she took the elevator to the basement and stood in front of the Burger Studio kiosk. Nothing interested her. She cranked her head from side to side to ease the tension and cranked it again.

"Looks like a bad stiff neck." Cate turned to see Jack Ross with an avuncular smile.

"It's the worst I've had in a long time."

"Liz used to get them. She hated them."

"I know why."

"I'm sorry you're uncomfortable. Looks like we both need food, and you need a break. How about burgers and beer at the Republic?"

"I should probably accept your offer. Jeff tells me I don't excel at spontaneity."

"What would he say if he were here?"

"He'd tell me to go. Enjoy a good burger, try a new craft beer." She laughed. "Okay, you're on. I'll get a coat and meet you at the front door in five. Are you going up?"

"A sweater and sports jacket work for me."

"What am I doing in a place where the upper forties feel like a heat wave?"

"The problem is, you're from St Louis, and I was born here. See you in five."

As they left the campus, Jack asked what was bothering her.

"I've been working all morning on a course aimed at graduates and undergraduates who want to learn about leadership, a summer course that the dean requested, and I can't figure out how to pitch it. It's the kind of problem I used to solve in my sleep."

"When your life was simpler?"

"I guess."

"With that kind of course, undergraduate or graduate doesn't matter. Decide what you want to teach and make electives available for those who want a challenge."

"Thanks. It sounds easy when you say it."

"Don't mention it," Jack grinned. "Next time, it might be me who needs the help."

"That's a generous thing to say."

Discreetly, Cate appraised Jack as they walked. She liked to tease him about his studied casualness but never in front of others. The laced gray Birkenstocks made her smile.

At a high-top table near the window, he ordered a pint of Surly Furious and the duck burger and recommended it to Cate. "You said Jeff would want you to try a good craft beer. Have you had Fulton Lonely Blonde?"

"I have, and I like it. For the beer, I'll stay with what I know, but I will try the duck burger."

"Not a beer you haven't tried?"

"That's as much adventure as I can handle. Hope you're not disappointed in me."

"Of course not."

"Good. Tell me about Japan," said Cate.

Jack laughed and answered eagerly.

"Turns out, Fukushima exemplifies how national culture drives government and business." He spoke with enthusiasm, his eyebrows in constant motion. "The independent commission that studied the Fukushima tragedy made use of our work. They blamed the disaster on

Japanese culture—deference to authority, reflexive obedience, loyalty to groups, shared social goals, and insularity. Those qualities drove Japan's postwar economic miracle. But they went off the rails when government and industry pursued energy security with the same unified purpose, ignoring the lessons of Three Mile Island and Chernobyl."

The waiter delivered the food and beer. They clinked glasses and drank.

"From what I've read, the crisis continues. There's contamination of soil, water, and fish."

"Exactly. What we're studying now is Japan's capacity to respond."

"I'm glad the sabbatical was so productive."

"I had a better winter than yours," said Jack. "How are you and the kids doing, and what's new with Jeff?"

Cate, who'd been leaning forward, sat back and exhaled. "He's been home for two and a half months, and we've settled into a routine. He's not the same, although his treatment team tries to be optimistic."

"It must be hard on Kayla and Ben."

"For sure, especially Ben. He was very anxious, but he's doing better."

"Good. And you?"

"I have to manage the home, direct his life, and keep the kids on track. I'm too busy to think about myself."

"Not to mention your thriving career."

"That keeps me going. That and the kids. I love what I do."

"I remember that feeling. When Liz was dying, I had to rely on work for stability. My kids were adults, so I didn't have to worry about them. Perhaps that made me lonelier."

"I miss Jeff's companionship, but I think you're right about the kids. It's good to have them, and Mandy helps a lot. Is it okay to ask how she's doing with you?"

"She's doing excellent work. Supervising her senior project is a pleasure. I can't thank you and Rosie enough for recommending me."

"Mandy and Rosie. Jeff called them the dynamite sisters." Cate took a gulp of beer and looked around. "You know, when I first came here a dozen years ago, this was Sgt. Preston's."

"I remember. Sgt. Preston's had great sandwiches, but the food got pretty grizzly at the end. Liz and I stopped going except to share fishbowl cocktails with friends before a Gopher's game. By the time the Republic opened, Liz was too sick to enjoy it." He coughed, and Cate thought his eyes grew moist. "Sixteen months," he said. "She died on the first day of December. She was fifty-eight and I was fifty-nine."

"Way too young."

"Liz was a senior at Princeton and applying to grad school in economics when we met. After we got engaged, she decided to stay at home. It was a huge mistake."

"Wow. At a time of women's lib."

"She and her family were old school. Still, skipping grad school was her dying regret. I should have encouraged her career. Maybe that's why I encourage yours."

"You miss her a lot, don't you?"

"Liz and I had a long time to talk about her death. She made me promise to live my life, but sometimes it's not so easy."

"Living a life can be very hard." Cate wiped a tear. "I can't talk with Jeff about his condition."

"That must feel very lonely. For both of you."

"I don't think Jeff can feel lonely. I wish he could; that would mean progress."

As they walked back to the university, Jack asked how Jeff managed alone all day.

"For the first six weeks after discharge, when it wasn't safe for him to leave the house alone or to use kitchen knives or the stove without help, he needed supervision 24/7. Now, on the days he's not at Sister Kenny, except when friends visit, he sits in front of the TV. He makes simple things like soup from a can, or I leave him a lunch."

"How often is Mandy there?"

"Several afternoons a week. She walks with him outside, pushes him to exercise, or makes him converse. She does have to work, even when the kids are there."

"She gets a lot done."

“It’s funny to think of Mandy in my house working on a project she does with you,” said Cate.

“It’s a nice connection.” Jack laughed. “I was thinking about that run we talked about, along the river. It’s a beautiful area with many ways to vary the run and lots of good places for a quick lunch afterwards.”

“I’ve been running in the Fieldhouse in the late morning.”

“I was thinking late afternoon, and you could go straight home. If you prefer midday and need a shower, you’re welcome to come upstairs and use mine.”

It seemed to Cate like a reasonable offer. She’d been to Jack’s condo many times in the past for dinner parties and faculty gatherings, the last time over a year and a half ago when Liz was alive. Cate checked her iPhone calendar, and they scheduled a run. Then they walked to their separate offices.

CHAPTER FORTY-ONE:

May

For Jeff, too much stimulation overwhelmed, but some remained essential. Scott and Meg had suggested Mother's Day brunch at the Arboretum, and Cate decided to risk it—a place busy but familiar. Brunch would be easy with friends present to occupy Jeff. Scott had made the reservations with Jeff conferenced into the call.

The large room at the visitor center was filled with spring flowers—crocuses, daffodils, tulips, brilliant azaleas, and white snowdrops—and a long table held a sumptuous spread of food. The moms and kids passed through the line and filled their plates with frittatas, Applewood-smoked bacon, pork sausage, and pastries. Then Scott shepherded Jeff through the line, and they returned with shrimp scampi, vegetables, and fruit. "Hey, you guys chose the healthy stuff," said Meg.

"I followed Jeff's lead," said Scott, "but if I hadn't intervened, he would've overflowed his plate. He kept piling it on."

"He's still learning to pace himself," said Cate.

Jeff was already chewing, looking only at his plate.

"At least the commotion doesn't bother him," said Meg.

"It probably does. That's why he narrows his focus," said Cate.

"Happy Mother's Day to the mothers among us," said Scott. Kayla nudged her dad.

"Oh, Happy Mother's Day," said Jeff.

"Thanks for making it special, honey," said Cate.

When everyone was stuffed, they left the café for the outdoors. Away from the clamor, Jeff grew more animated. The Arboretum had thirty-five thousand tulips, half of them in bloom, and he warmed to their vibrant colors. They left the tulips and wandered through the Arboretum's quiet, defined spaces—the rock garden with creeping phlox, the bog with native lady slipper orchids, the wildflower garden with trilliums and Johnny jump-ups—and Cate hooked Jeff's arm. Awkwardly, he kissed Cate's cheek.

"Nice kiss," said Kayla. Cate laughed at Jeff's bemused expression.

As they climbed into Meg and Scott's van for the three-mile drive, Jeff pulled once more into himself. "Jeff, you love the Arboretum, and we often take this drive—so quiet and peaceful, and always different," said Cate.

"You love it, too," said Jeff, who seemed to come alive when they reached the magnolias and crabapple trees, white to pink to prairie fire red.

"We hit these at the perfect time!" said Meg.

"We sure did," said Scott.

"Thanks for taking us here, guys," said Cate. She took Jeff's hand. He covered it and smiled.

They exited the drive and headed to the spring plant sale, where Meg bought astilbe and columbine for her shaded backyard and native Minnesota ostrich ferns known for delicious fiddleheads. Jeff was drawn again to tulips. Cate, who'd not gardened for years, decided to plant some bulbs next fall, but she wanted color now. Jeff and the kids picked out budding tulips by looking at pictures of what they'd become. Kayla and Ben loved the Prince family of tulips, White Prince, Candy Prince, and Purple Rain—white, soft and deep purple—and Cate included some of those.

At home, Cate stored the bulbs in a dark, cool corner of the basement and arranged the budding tulips on the patio. "Tulips," said Jeff. "We're gonna have tulips.

CHAPTER FORTY-TWO:

Late May

Sometimes it felt like teaching a slow child; other times, Jeff's improvement, however slight, pulled her forward. Cate tried to engage him in the morning when he was fresh and most alert, and she had more patience. "Jeff, what do you want to work on today?"

"I'm too tired in the evening to have fun with kids."

"Do you know you're grumpy too?"

"Okay, tired and grumpy."

"That's a good beginning, Mr. Grumpy," said Cate, smiling. Jeff returned the grin. Cate hesitated, but she wanted to know. "Why did you smile?"

"Because you did."

"Not because I called you Mr. Grumpy?"

"I'm not Mr. Grumpy. I'm Jeff."

Cate looked away. She took a sip of tea, then another, and crossed her arms. "Okay, let's keep working. When do you start to notice that you're tired and grumpy?"

"After a while."

"When you're with the kids?"

"Yes." He scratched his chin.

"Are you sure that's right?"

"No. I know it now."

"That means you can anticipate, honey. It means you're getting better." Jeff responded with a yawn. Cate gripped his wrist. "Stay with it, Jeff, and tell me why it matters. You can do this."

"I want to have fun. They do too."

"Good." Cate leaned toward him. "What would help you do that?"

Jeff narrowed his eyes in thought. "An afternoon nap?"

"What do you think?"

"Yes, a nap, and if I'm irritable, I could take a break."

"All right!" Cate thumped his shoulder. She studied his face, hoping for emotion, but saw none. No satisfaction, no distress. She pushed her chair away from the table. "Okay, let's take a five-minute break." She boiled water for tea and watched Jeff make a cup of coffee with the Keurig, a multistep process he could now accomplish on his own. "Read that Keurig screen, honey. It tells you to enjoy the coffee."

"I will enjoy it," he said, reading the screen without a trace of irony. Cate set her jaw.

"Ready?" Jeff nodded. "Before we stopped, we were working on what makes you tired and grumpy in the evenings." She handed him what Lori called the *Multi-Factor Worksheet* and pointed to the first box.

"Brain factors," Jeff read.

"That's the easy one, isn't it?"

"My brain injury."

"Write that down. Now, what about that injury?"

"I think slowly."

"And?"

"I can't handle too much at once."

"Good." He wrote those down. Cate paused, allowing him to reflect.

"Okay, let's go to the next box." Under *personal factors*, with Cate's help, he wrote *too tired to concentrate, and headache.* "And that makes you feel how?" He added *mixed up, grumpy, and discouraged.*

Cate stood and stretched. Jeff did the same.

"Okay, you're on a roll, honey, and we're almost done. The last box said *situational factors.* Jeff wrote *too much noise and trying to do too much at once.*

"Nice work. The idea is that all of these factors—*brain, personal and situational*—interact. That's what this worksheet is all about.

They'd finished, but Jeff looked restless, which made Cate tense. "Would you like to take a walk before I go to work?" Jeff nodded. They donned light jackets. The morning was sunny and warm, and they strolled, at first stiffly, then with an easier pace, hand in hand. They walked a half mile, and by the time they returned to the house, their hands were gently swinging.

* * *

Later that day, Cate had lunch with Meg in a secluded corner of the Campus Club and talked about the morning. "It's heartening and disheartening," said Cate. "He's making progress, but we barely scratch the surface."

"He knows he gets tired. That's good."

"I can help him list factors that contribute, but he doesn't appreciate the interactions. It feels like I make all my effort. What I get back is a pale reflection of my energy." Cate watched her fingers curl around the glass of wine, lift the cup, and start to move the cup toward her lips. She stopped, the glass in midair. "Shit, I'm watching myself drink wine, breaking it into steps."

Meg laughed. "See, you've acquired a new skill. Now tell me how you feel, what contributes, and how the factors interact?"

"Haha," said Cate, but she finished the wine with gusto.

On the way back to their offices, they stopped above the river to look north toward the Mississippi headwaters. "You do love this river," said Meg.

"It's always there, always flowing."

"I love that you love this river."

"Thanks. I love its strength. Its reliability."

Ninety days, Cate thought. "You know, a drop of rain that fell in Itasca on the day of Jeff's accident reached the ocean almost three months ago," said Cate. "If I could time Jeff's recovery by a succession of drops, each trip one segment of recovery, he's about to finish the second segment."

"Wow. Six months."

"In a week."

With an appreciative glance at the river, Cate took Meg's arm, and they marched arm in arm until their paths diverged.

* * *

That evening, Cate appraised Jeff as he stepped from the shower and dried himself. Without his usual tan, the wrinkled scar on his left shoulder blended easily into his skin. He looked good, despite loss of muscle and fat, and Cate felt a tingling between her thighs, still familiar although six months had passed since the night before Jeff's accident and the warmth of the next morning. Since the night of discharge, when an attempt at intimacy left her dispirited and overwhelmed, she had avoided sex except for an occasional hug and a brush of lips. Several times, she'd touched herself in the shower, a pleasurable release, but she preferred shared arousal, the sensual rubbing of bodies. Jeff reached for his pajamas. "Don't do that," said Cate.

"Do what?"

"Put those on."

"Why not?"

His question sent Cate into her head, where she didn't want to be. The doctors had warned that loss of sexual desire was common with frontal lobe brain injuries. It might not work, but it was the right time to try once more. Cate touched her thighs, and the tingling increased.

"Watch," she said. She looked steadily at Jeff as she removed her nightgown, her nipples hard and erect. He made no move toward her. She touched his lips with her fingers, searching for arousal, but saw none.

"Let's hug like we used to." She pressed her body against his, took his hands, and put them just behind her waist. "Reach around and put your hands on my back." She put her arms around him to show him and squeezed. He clutched her clumsily.

With a sigh, she released him and motioned to the bed. He sat, and she perched beside him. "Honey, I want to make love, do you?" He nodded as if he knew what she expected. She decided to risk the intimacy of a kiss, put her hand on his chin, turned his head gently, brushed her lips against his, and then pressed firmly. She parted her lips and pressed her tongue between his lips until they parted, and their tongues touched. His lips grew firm, and his tongue began to probe. His breath quickened, and so did hers. But Jeff seemed to lose interest and pulled back.

They sat, legs touching, but her nipples had softened. She trudged to the bathroom and took a long drink of cold water.

"Okay, honey. Let's try this. Lie on your side facing me." She kissed his face, his neck, and shoulders, gently rubbed her fingernails along his back and again kissed his lips. He kissed back. She moved her lips to his chest and sides and kissed his legs from ankles to thighs. She returned to his lips and hugged him. He pushed his body against hers.

"Here. Touch me." She took his hand and placed it on her breast. He held it there until she showed him how to stroke her. A memory sparked, and he leaned down to kiss her breasts, tickling her nipples gently with his tongue. She bent her head back and moaned softly. He lifted his head to look at her. "Don't stop," she said. Firmly, she pushed his head back against her breasts. With the other hand, she touched his thighs, stoked his scrotum, and massaged his penis, which had barely hardened.

"Touch me here," she said, guiding his hand. As she grew wet, she continued to stroke his penis, rolling it rhythmically between her thumb and fingers, and slowly it came alive. She pulled back and smiled at him, still stroking. They kissed, and this time he pressed firmly, with urgency. His hips began to move, like an animal coming alive, remembering what to do. He was breathing quickly now. Cate was wet, throbbing with desire. Yet she yearned for closeness and intimacy, more than release, and she did not feel it.

Finally, as they kissed and touched, she guided him inside her, and they moved, the length of their bodies touching, their hips thrusting with shared urgency, every inch of skin electric until they exploded in unison.

They lay together, panting. Jeff grew soft, still inside her, but neither pulled back. She kissed his neck, enjoying the taste of his sweat.

Finally, flushed and spent, they lay facing each other. “Jeff, I love you, I love you so much.” She wanted to love him, to feel the pleasure of intimacy.

One of Jeff’s arms rested against his chest, between them, and his expression grew flat. He closed his eyes and breathed with the rhythm of sleep.

Tears filled Cate’s eyes.

She tried to rest but could not sleep. She pulled the covers over Jeff and descended to the kitchen, made herself a cup of chamomile tea, and sat in the family room watching the black hearth where a fire should burn, until she fell asleep on the couch.

When she awoke, the morning sun shined through the family room windows.

CHAPTER FORTY-THREE:

Early June

After an hour of research at the worktable in her university office, Cate moved to the Bordeaux chair and leaned back, enjoying its comfort. She opened her iPhone to yesterday's family pictures. Because the day had been dark and cloudy with a stiff breeze and chance of rain, chilly enough to require spring jackets, few had chosen that day to picnic. The children loved the adventure—everyone zipped up, burgers cooking on the hibachi, smoke condensing above the charcoal, Jeff helping to cook.

They'd asked a passerby to snap a family photo, which turned out to be a striking image, Jeff tall in the center of the blanket, the children and Cate leaning toward him like a medieval painting, Jeff exalted, detached, sublime, an icon from a different world. The image lingered as she stood and stretched and gazed at the Bordeaux chair. She turned her back to the chair and returned to the worktable.

Cate opened her computer and immersed herself in the summer leadership course that would begin tomorrow. Once the conversation with Jack had freed her imagination, she decided to make it a seminar rather than a series of lectures. She visualized the classroom, placing herself in front of students, involving them, inviting curiosity. Jeff used to say that every class was an opportunity to build community, and that was how she approached teaching.

She'd begin the first day with four slides, the only slides she'd use: first a picture of Mandela, then a second slide with ten words and phrases that described him—courage, perseverance, optimism, resilience, commitment, creativity, humor, compassion, forgiveness, the capacity to inspire.

After that came a picture of Bob Dylan and a final slide with more descriptors. Original, iconoclastic, lyrical, poetic, and a question: what made Dylan so influential?

Then, with the four slides projected together on the screen, Cate would ask the students to debate the qualities of transformative leaders and ideas. That discussion would fill the first day.

As homework, she'd ask them to think about leaders they had admired and known personally, describe them in writing, and prepare to discuss in class the qualities that made them effective. That would fill the second day.

Thereafter, the students would explore what ideas inspired them, how they might mobilize people toward a shared goal, what made that goal worthwhile, and what elements of a goal might make it aspirational. She'd get them talking to each other, challenging and encouraging one another. By the end of the class, they would each, in their own way, be leaders.

She was still smiling when Jennifer knocked on her door. They'd scheduled a meeting with Rosie to review the galley proof of the symposium Proceedings, but Jen arrived early.

"I wanted to catch you before we meet with Rosie," said Jennifer.

"What's up?"

"Bette," the department chair, "tried to reach you, but had to leave and asked me to tell you that your promotion to full professor was approved!"

"Hey, thanks," said Cate, accepting Jennifer's congratulatory hug.

Shortly thereafter, Rosie arrived. They'd read through the proofs, so it took only a few minutes to approve the Proceedings and dispatch them to the publisher. They hoped for a quick release: transformational leadership was a fast-moving topic in academia.

As she was seated at her desk, Cate's gaze fell on the empty bottle of Saint-Emilion Grand Cru. She retrieved it, placed it on the wine-red executive desk chair, and savored the moment when Jeff, excited and proud, had given them to her to celebrate her last promotion. She left the wine bottle resting on its side in the middle of the chair and stood looking out the window toward the Mississippi. In winter, she could see a trace of the river between the brick buildings, but in June, luxuriant trees blocked her view. With a sigh, she returned to the worktable.

After another hour, glancing from time to time at the wine bottle nestled in the chair, the alarm on Cate's iPhone chimed. She changed into running gear and drove to the Stone Arch Bridge, which crossed the Mississippi near the Guthrie Theater, to run with Jack. They'd been running along the river trails more or less weekly for the past few weeks, always at the end of a day, after which she'd head home to shower and dress. Today, they planned a late morning run, a change of pace for both, and lunch at the Mill City Museum, where she could eat in running gear and shower later at the University Fieldhouse or end the day at home.

"Ready?" asked Jack.

"Let's get going. It's a little nippy." Cate had goosebumps, more than she usually had with a gentle chill.

"If you're cold, let's run first and talk later. Are you up to three or four miles?"

"You bet."

They ran at an easy pace across the Stone Arch Bridge and paused on the other end, standing close, to watch a barge rise slowly in the lock as the Mississippi tumbled over St. Anthony Falls. Cate shivered and rubbed her arms to chase away the gooseflesh. "Did you know they're closing this lock, after fifty years of river navigation, to keep Asian carp from the upper river? It's the end of an era," said Jack.

"I read about that," said Cate. "Without the Mississippi, there wouldn't be a Minneapolis."

"That's for sure. They built sawmills and flour mills here to use the power of the falls." Jack looked at Cate, who gave a slight nod, and they resumed, jogging left off the bridge onto Main Street, then down a narrow street onto Nicollet Island. Jack pointed at the huge Grain Belt beer sign, prominent in iconic pictures of Minneapolis at night, listed on the National Register of Historic Places. "I can see this sign from my condo," he said, "and I just read that Schell Brewing and the city are talking about relighting it."

"Let's stop for a minute. My heart is racing."

"We usually run faster than this."

"I know, and it's cold, but I need to stop." Cate zipped up her jacket, crossed her arms and slapped her shoulders to warm herself. Once again, they took off, zigzagging through the north end of the island, past historic homes tucked away from the concrete jungle that surrounded it, continued north off the island, turned right back toward Main Street, ran at top speed for the last leg of the run, and returned to the Stone Arch Bridge, a clockwise circuit of around four miles. They walked across the bridge toward Jack's condo, found a bench, and rested.

"Finally, I'm warm. Even sweaty, probably too much for lunch at the museum."

"You'll be fine." Jack grinned. "Now that you're warm, I get to ask about your day."

"It's been a perfect morning." She described the course that would start tomorrow and the Proceedings dispatched to the editor.

"There's something else, because you're smiling," said Jack.

"Just before I left to come here, I found out that my promotion was approved."

"That's wonderful! If you'd like to come upstairs, I'll crack open a good bottle of wine to toast your promotion before lunch."

"That's tempting."

"If you'll be more comfortable, you can shower and change first. There's plenty of privacy."

"Why not? I could use a glass of wine." They walked to Cate's car to fetch her backpack and change of clothes, then to his condo that stood near the base of the bridge, and they took the elevator to Jack's large top-floor apartment, which looked the same as Cate recalled. She remembered the large picture window that overlooked the Stone Arch

Bridge, the beautiful views to the east and northwest past Nicollet Island, and the outdated 1990s décor that traditional Liz still favored in 2004 when they bought and furnished the apartment, the living room hunter green and burgundy with damask wallpaper and track lighting, made interesting by Japanese furniture and accent pieces purchased over the years on trips to Japan and elsewhere. Bird and floral prints covered the walls in the rest of the apartment, and the kitchen was completely white.

Jack pointed out the Grain Belt sign and the route they'd run. "Bathroom's that way." He gestured down the hall. "If a cabernet's okay, I've got a nice one."

"I love a good cabernet."

In the bathroom, Cate undressed and spotted a full-length mirror that must have been Liz's. Her body had not lost its tone, thanks to gymnastics with Kayla and an occasional run. *C'mon, Cate,* she told herself. *You have a mirror at home.* When she returned to the living room, dressed, Jack stood looking out the window, also freshly showered, in a honey-brown shirt flecked with amber and olive.

"Nice shirt, Jack. Matches your hazel eyes."

"Birthday present from Liz. She found them online and bought me half a dozen similar to this. You look pretty good yourself." The table in front of the couch held two wine glasses, a bottle of cabernet, crackers, and an array of cheeses.

"Do you usually keep cheeses on hand?"

"I do, in case I have friends over. If they're not eaten, I bring them to the break room at work. Sorry I don't have red grapes to go with them."

"Wine and cheese are plenty." Cate spread a soft cheese on a cracker and ate it. "Saint-André?"

"Good palate." Jack poured the wine. "This cabernet is from a wine-loving friend in California." Jack handed her a glass and raised his. "To the new Professor and a career of continued success."

"To my mentor, colleague, and friend." They clinked glasses and sipped. "Wow, this wine is excellent. Wine, cheese, and a view. You know how to live."

"The view is even better from the terrace." Cate had forgotten that Jack's apartment was a penthouse. They climbed the stairs to an open space with chairs and a table, an umbrella, and an even better panorama. Jack stood close enough for Cate to smell the wine on his breath, which reminded her of the empty wine bottle lying in her office on the wine-red chair. She pushed away that thought.

"This is like a piece of heaven."

"Liz and I used to spend a lot of time up here, but now I mainly stay below."

"It's beautiful downstairs, too."

"It needs refreshing, but you know what I mean. From what you've told me about Jeff's injury, in a way, you've lost someone too."

"That's true." Cate stared into the horizon. Jack touched her arm, and warmth from his touch made her quiver as she turned her head to look at Jack. "But this is your place. I should be consoling you."

"My loss was eighteen months ago. I'm adjusting. Yours continues to evolve."

"You've always understood that. You and Meg."

"I've always liked Meg. She's a good person."

"Meg's not here right now." Cate pivoted so that her whole body faced Jack, aware that she had accepted the invitation to his apartment with more eagerness than caution. She'd wanted to kiss Jack for a long time. For six months, she'd experienced no soothing touch from Jeff, no physical affection; she could feel the struggle within her, hunger and need battling loyalty and devotion. She knew that Jack liked her. She knew that Jack, proper and considerate, would never make an advance. It occurred to her that it would be easier to succumb than initiate, but the thought annoyed her. Cate was not sure what she wanted, but it was up to her to decide.

Cate took a half step toward him, and her breath quickened. "It must be hard without Liz."

"It's very hard." Jack held his ground.

But Cate flinched. "Let's go downstairs," she said, stepping back. Jack led the way, and he settled on the couch, framed by the picture window and the horizon. Cate took the chair opposite him but didn't try to hide her desire; she sat, watching the tension build, knowing they both felt it.

"Cate," he said softly, "we're both lonely, but I don't want to jeopardize our friendship."

"Neither do I. But maybe we can change it." Her eyes held his and this time didn't falter as she moved to the couch.

"I don't know if this is a good idea," he said.

"I'd like to try and see where it goes. You did invite me to your apartment."

"I hesitated. Because I like you, and I don't want anybody to get hurt. What about Jeff?"

"I love Jeff, and hurting him is the last thing I want, but part of him is missing and I've never felt so alone."

"Cate, I'm not sure how to say this, but I don't want to be your Band-Aid, and I don't want you to be mine."

"I like you, and I know you like me. That's not a Band-Aid. It's a relationship." She put one hand beneath his chin, and they looked at each other for several seconds before they kissed. Their lips parted, and the kiss grew more intense. Cate's blouse was unbuttoned, and Jack's shirt pulled up before Cate spoke again. "Wouldn't we be more comfortable in the bedroom?" she whispered.

"Are you sure?"

"Can't you tell?" She touched his shoulder with her fingers and moved them slowly down his arm. When her fingers reached his hand, he took it and led her to the bedroom.

* * *

To Cate's surprise, she felt relaxed and comfortable. "Are you hungry?" asked Jack.

"Not anymore," she said, her voice tender. They sat in the living room, wearing robes, Jack in beige terrycloth, Cate in Jack's black silk robe. Jack didn't say, but Cate guessed it was a gift from Liz. Jack grinned and pointed to the cheese.

"We can have that, or we can still go to lunch."

"This is fine, even without the grapes."

"Cate," Jack hesitated, his manner gentle but serious. "I didn't expect the run to end like this. This is very new to me."

"It's new to me too." Cate squinted at the flowing river. "I enjoy spending time with you."

"I enjoy it too …" He hesitated.

"I've never seen you at a loss for words before," said Cate with a grin.

"I want to get this right, so we stay comfortable with each other." His tone was soft and serious.

"Like being discreet at work?"

"That part shouldn't be difficult if we're intentional about it. What about Jeff?"

"You mean me and Jeff?"

"Yes. That's what I really want to know. Lord knows I wish him well."

"He'll be there, but he won't have much capacity for emotion."

Cate studied Jack. She understood that people found him intimidating—he could use his intellect to slice with sardonic precision—yet she had always found him kind and gentle.

"You know I could never leave him. I wouldn't."

"I'm glad to hear that, even though it also makes me sad. It preserves my good opinion of you." He poured some wine and sipped. "What's he like now?"

"It's hard to describe. I had a nightmare the other night that Jeff was a zombie, lifeless, a body without a soul. It's not that bad, but there's no warmth or affection." Cate stared at the waterfall.

"I think of Jeff as warm and witty."

"He was. That's what's so painful, knowing that part of him is gone. You know, I have no idea what he feels; he can't tell me, so I have to figure it out from his behavior. The only emotion he shows is irritability when he's stressed or tired."

"After six months?"

"Almost to the day, which the doctors say is an important milestone because improvement slows after that. There will be much slower improvement in the next six months, even less in the year after that; recovery is a two-year process with most of it early." She shook her head with an air of resignation. "They say his ability to function will likely get better. How much is anyone's guess, but the personality change, the apathy, the inertness is not likely to improve, although they keep telling me there might be pleasant surprises."

Jack inclined his head and listened. He asked about the kids, and Cate responded that Ben needed a little help, but both were resilient.

"There's another part of this. Jeff's work. We visited his lab briefly, where his partner keeps the business going. Maybe he'll try in a few months, but it's doubtful he can do anything productive."

"Everything's on your shoulders."

"We have twelve years of history and a family, but I doubt we'll ever be able to have a real relationship. Not anymore. That's why I need love in my life, the kind that offers companionship."

"I understand that. It's been a year and a half since Liz died, and it looks like I'm ready to try again."

"Jack, I don't want to stand in your way. Maybe you'll meet someone."

"I just did." Jack grinned, his smile both playful and kind. "I think we can do this and not lose respect for each other or for ourselves. That's important to me."

"It is to me too."

"What are you going to do after this?"

"I'm going back to the office because work is my solace. You might find this amusing, but I want this to feel like a normal day, except that I hope *you* are not going back to the office. I need a day before I can run into you at the university and keep a straight face."

She brushed Jack's lips, dressed in the bathroom, and left for her office, where a wine-red chair and an empty bottle waited.

CHAPTER FORTY-FOUR:

Early August

Cate and Jeff loved the Angry Trout in Grand Marais, a café and restaurant on the edge of Lake Superior on Minnesota's North Shore, accessible by land or by boat from the picturesque harbor. As they waited for their order on the patio, a small catboat arrived at the end of the dock with a family of four that made Cate think of Kayla and Ben, who usually vacationed with them. It was a gorgeous day and a lovely setting, yet Cate's mood was bittersweet. Before the accident, they'd planned a family camping trip into the Boundary Waters that had morphed into a five-day vacation for the two of them, a trip to get away as a couple, a suggestion from Meg and Scott, who offered to watch the kids.

Cate gazed past the catboat at the harbor, sailboats on buoys in the cove, blue waves crashing against the lighthouse at the end of the long, curved jetty that protected the harbor, sailboats with shimmering white sails beyond the jetty, and further out a larger sloop with rust-red sails made full by the brisk wind. Cate and Jeff had discovered Grand Marais eleven years ago, two months after their first anniversary, when they headed north for a vacation. Since then, they'd come every summer to the picturesque village and to the Gunflint Lodge an hour northwest, heading inland along the Gunflint Trail, first as a couple for camping, canoeing, hiking, and fishing in the Boundary Waters, leaving the kids with grandparents, then as a family to enjoy the village, lodge, lake, and woods. They'd even visited twice between Christmas and New Year's Day, most recently a year and a half ago, to snowmobile and cross-country ski with the kids.

Scott had suggested that they leave Thursday morning and return Monday to avoid weekend traffic. During the almost five-hour drive, the first time Cate had driven the entire way, she kept up the chatter, and Jeff responded most of the time. In two weeks, Jeff would take a driving test at the Courage Center. Cate wondered if he'd pass.

Seated at the restaurant, Cate tried to anticipate four nights at the Gunflint Lodge, time to sit, walk in the woods, and enjoy the water, no shuttle this time to the Boundary Waters entry point, and no camping. Just the quiet knotty pine cabin place, a king-size bed, and a kitchen that would go unused in favor of meals in the lodge.

"Do you remember the first time you brought me up north?" asked Cate. Cate had never camped, let alone in a wilderness, and Jeff talked her into a canoe trip and two nights in the Boundary Waters. The idea of cooking on a campfire and sleeping under the stars held no appeal for Cate, who feared getting lost and thought they should hire a guide, but Jeff said he'd been camping in the Boundary Waters since he was a child. It proved to be the best vacation of Cate's life, just the two of them, no other campers seen or heard, no motors, no pollution, alone to enjoy wilderness forests, glacial lakes, brilliant sunsets, dark nights filled with stars, and the most intense and profound quiet Cate had ever experienced.

"Before setting out, we sat on this very deck, and you teased me about getting lost. I almost told you to take that trip and shove it." She took his hand and held it. "Then you made it sound romantic, the two of us on the edge of a million acres of remote woods and water, ungodly beautiful, primitive and unspoiled."

"I remember. You were scared, and I teased you."

"I loved that trip and all the ones that followed. This time, honey, we won't be camping. We'll hike and canoe, but only on the lake." She squeezed Jeff's hand and smiled. "No portages this year."

"Where will we sleep?"

"In the lodge," said Cate. "We'll eat there too. I won't get to eat your campfire cooking."

"Too bad," he said. The words felt right, but his voice was as flat as a breeze-free lake. She watched the sailboats and the wind.

"Look at the waves lashing against the lighthouse," she said. "I love it when Lake Superior shows its power." They savored the fresh lake air and the last bites of grilled whitefish.

"Ready to go?" asked Cate, and Jeff nodded. It would take an hour to drive the forty-three miles to the lodge, with plenty of time to hike or canoe, or relax before dinner.

* * *

Cate moved gingerly through the pitch-black night, a half step in front of Jeff, holding his hand, leading him up the hill, as her feet groped for purchase on the rocky path, trying to feel pebbles through her walking shoes. Sweat trickled down her neck as she pointed out the path to Jeff, worried that he might fall, following a guide from the Gunflint Lodge whom she could hear but not see, afraid that this guided midnight hike through a moonless night had been a mistake. Gradually, after about five minutes, Cate began to trust her feet and settled into a steady meditative gait, contemplating the sounds of the black forest. Owls hooted, birds chirped, and soft rustling underbrush confirmed that small animals kept them company in the cool night air. "Are you okay, Jeff?"

"Fine."

They reached a clearing and stopped. With eyes dilated to accommodate the dark, Cate could, with effort, see the forest and sense it drop away somewhere in front of them. Cate followed the guide's finger to Gunflint Lake. No moon glinted on the water; there was only the impression of a flat surface beyond the trees as she held Jeff's hand and listened to the night. With the lake as background, Cate could make out the guide and several others. From the direction of the flat surface, a loon wailed and another answered.

"If you haven't been here during the day, it's worth the hike, especially now that you've experienced it at night," said the guide.

Cate gave Jeff's hand a squeeze. "We know this trail. Let's come back after breakfast." He squeezed in affirmation.

"We'll take a different route back to the lodge," said the guide. "It's hillier, with sharp curves." Cate continued to trust her feet, alert to the sound of Jeff's muted steps as cicadas hummed and clicked in the background. Around a curve, something large moved a couple of yards in front of them; a buck with a huge rack faded like a shadow into the woods. "That's a treat," said the guide. "They don't usually get so close."

Halfway down the hill, the guide paused. "Be very still and listen for a while." He pointed out the staccato notes of the saw-whet owl, the raspy bark of a distant fox, the breeze murmuring through pines, and from the lake behind them, the yodel of a male loon. They finished the walk, alive to the sounds of the north woods.

Back in the lodge, Jeff wanted to stop at the bar, which was about to close. "Honey, you haven't had any alcohol since the accident."

"A beer's okay," said Jeff, and ordered a pint of Moose Drool.

"Let's share it." Jeff agreed. Cate asked for a second glass, and they split the pint of brown ale. The beer seemed to relax him, with no ill effects. They returned to the cabin, showered, and crawled into bed close to one in the morning.

It was late, a reason to go right to sleep. But this was supposed to be a honeymoon of sorts, and they had not had intercourse since the accident, except the one time. Sometimes, at home, Cate kissed his forehead, caressed the scar on his shoulder, or hugged his still-handsome body, and sometimes he hugged her back; usually, Jeff fell instantly asleep, and Cate felt more relief than disappointment, especially in the past two months, when Jack Ross had begun to fill that void.

She didn't want to think of Jack, but he kept intruding. It helped that Jack remained considerate and discreet, that they communicated well, liked and understood each other, and that Meg was supportive of the relationship with Jack. Meg understood Cate's need for warmth and attachment, the depth of loneliness that Cate experienced, the importance of intimacy; she even suggested that the relationship with

Jack, if it reduced Cate's despair, would help her care more effectively for Jeff. If that relationship helped Cate to keep her family intact, then it was worth the emotional dissonance, even if Cate thought about it as a double life.

Cate looked at Jeff, naked in the king-size bed, awake in the dim light. He smiled, and Cate thought she saw life in his eyes; she wanted life. She lay next to him and began to caress him. After a while, he caressed her too, as if she had touched something primitive and deep, awakened some part of him from hibernation, and Cate began to feel her body respond. She kissed his mouth, and he kissed her back. He touched her breasts and kissed them. They hugged and kissed and touched until he was hard, and she was wet, although part of her felt numb. Neither spoke. No words. No expressions of love.

To her surprise, Jeff rolled her onto her back, suspended himself above her, and moved until he satisfied her before his own release. Yet the pleasure felt remote, as if her body were not her own. She was not surprised when Jeff withdrew, turned on his side, and slept.

Cate had hoped for love and intimacy. What she felt were loneliness and grief. And recognition—all that Jeff had lost—what she had not let herself accept.

She sobbed, looking at the sleeping form of the man she'd loved, still loved, would always love. The man who had gone missing. The man she would never leave. For her kids, for herself—for Jeff—she would make the best of the situation. That was the part that she could—she would—control.

She knew that the next morning would come, and what it would be. She also knew that some small part of her would continue to hope.

* * *

After a few hours of sleep, they went to breakfast early. Cate had to help Jeff order, as his capacities were uneven, unpredictable; sometimes, he couldn't make the easiest decision.

When they finished, Cate took Jeff's arm, and they found the path they'd taken the night before. They hiked up to the clearing where they'd stood holding hands and sat on a rustic bench. Cate, who'd learned to recognize the calls of songbirds over the years—whistling chickadees, flutelike thrushes, trilling warblers, chirping flycatchers, and harsh jays—identified them but couldn't spot them, even as she searched the trees. Beyond a railing in front of them, the forest dropped away as she remembered it, and the lake glistened in the sun. They spotted a loon, tiny in the distance, and listened to its wail echo with haunting clarity.

Jeff, more alert than usual despite the short sleep, pointed at a spot below them where the trees thinned. A shadow moved and an antlered buck, not as close as the one last night, vanished into the deep woods. "Good eyes," said Cate.

They walked back to the lodge and down to Gunflint Lake, took paddles, and pushed a canoe into the water. Jeff took the rear and kept their path straight. Cate turned, watched him execute a perfect J stroke, and guessed that he was responding to body memories. They paddled toward the center of the lake, where the water was blue and glassy and looked solid as a floor, but the lake was long and large, half in Canada and half in the United States. Just south of where the border might be, they stowed the paddles, and Cate could almost enjoy the moment, husband and wife on vacation.

When the sun grew hot, Cate pointed to the dock, and they started back toward the lodge.

Toward a new reality where Jeff would live his heartbreaking, muted life. With Cate, melancholic and resigned, determined to make it work. All of it.

CHAPTER FORTY-FIVE:

September

By mid-September, Cate had resumed her hectic schedule and the children had settled into school. The symposium Proceedings had appeared with favorable reviews and warm congratulations from Jack, although two weeks had passed with no time for Jack except a hurried lunch in the food court.

Three weeks earlier, Jeff had failed the Courage Center driving test. In the past week, following test recommendations, he'd started to drive for short periods during the day on quiet neighborhood streets with Cate beside him. Overall, Jeff progressed inch by sluggish inch. As he learned to use his logbook to bring assignments home each week, Cate reduced her attendance at Cognitive OT to once a month, yet Jeff continued to ignore homework unless prompted.

Twice Cate had driven Jeff to his lab and watched him walk around like a dog sniffing out territory once familiar, perturbed by slight changes initiated by his partner—his desk against a different wall, a freezer moved, a new lab bench. He tried, with the help of Bill, his partner, to do a few simple tasks, but made little effort. It didn't look like productive work was on Jeff's horizon, although Bill was willing to allow him to try. Perhaps he could work with farmers. To do that, he had to drive to farms.

On a Wednesday, Cate returned in the early afternoon to work at home, where she could be close to Jeff. As she entered the house, she checked her phone and found a text message from Bonnie that said Ben was back in class and doing fine.

"Jeff, do you know anything about a problem with Ben at school?"

"He was attacked."

Cate imagined a schoolyard fight.

"Attacked? For God's sake, why didn't you call me?"

"She said he was okay."

"Who?"

"The nurse."

"Do you know what happened?"

"An attack." Jeff seemed unperturbed.

With her heart pounding, Cate called the school nurse, who was not available. She asked for Bonnie, who told Cate that Ben had a mild panic attack, apparently precipitated by getting a question wrong when the teacher called on him. The nurse recognized what was happening, let Ben rest for twenty minutes in her office, comforted him, and sent him back to class. A few minutes later, when the nurse and Bonnie checked, he was unruffled and engaged in classwork.

"Has he had panic attacks before?" asked Bonnie.

"Not that I've observed. My sister used to get them, so I know what they are, and Ben's psychiatrist told me that he might have had mild ones. A big one didn't seem likely, so I didn't tell the school."

"That's okay. We managed. How are you doing?"

"Upset. Jeff said he was attacked."

"Who told him that?"

"The school nurse. At least that's what he heard."

"Uh-oh. It's a substitute nurse, and she didn't know about Jeff's injury. I'll make sure the nurses know to call you."

"The psychiatrist said Ben's medication should help panic attacks. I'll see if she has any suggestions. Now that I know Ben's okay, I'm more upset about Jeff. He wasn't at all concerned."

"Really? That surprises me."

"Me too." Cate thanked Bonnie, who promised to stay in touch, and turned to Jeff.

"Dammit, he wasn't attacked. He had a panic attack."

"She said he was okay."

"Jeff, get out your logbook and write this down. 'If the school calls about Ben or Kayla, I have to call Cate.' Write down *exactly* what I said." He did. "Okay, now read me what you wrote."

After that discussion, Cate retreated to her home office, talked to the psychiatrist's nurse, who promised to get back to her, and phoned Lori, Jeff's Cognitive OT therapist. Lori answered, and Cate described what had happened. "This feels new to me. How could he make that kind of mistake?"

"I understand your shock, but it's not really new. It's all part of his impaired judgment."

"How can that be? He talks, he smiles, he interacts. It looks like he's coming back."

"Think about what happened the other morning with the game." Jeff had started to play crazy eights with Ben at breakfast, even though it was time to leave for school, and didn't understand Cate's annoyance. "Or the problems with homework." Last visit, they discussed the way Jeff made errors on homework and thought Cate and Lori were making a big deal out of nothing. "This is all about judgment, and this time it mattered more than crazy eights or homework. I know it's hard to see and harder to accept, but it's the kind of problem that might persist."

"I keep hoping for more. It's been nine months."

"From time to time, you get a different glimpse of his disability. It's all part of the recovery process, and I know it's hard."

Cate ended the call. She felt like the tires of Jeff's recovery vehicle, the fuel for its engine. She wanted to steer it but could not get the wheel to turn.

Some months ago, Dr. Hunter had told her that Jeff would experience frustration and depression as he improved. The greater his awareness, the more his distress. This might be hard on their relationship, but his depression would reflect progress.

To the degree that Jeff did not improve, their relationship would be more like parent and child. She would be the one to experience distress and depression.

Cate thought about that as she sank into the couch, bone-weary. She had an hour to rest before Kayla and Ben got home from school. An hour to pull herself together.

* * *

That evening, determined to keep pushing Jeff toward recovery, to make it easier for him to resume driving and perhaps work, Cate searched the internet and found a dealer with a certified, pre-owned 2011 Toyota SUV, the same model as Jeff's old one, except that the color was navy blue instead of silver.

An actual vehicle, thought Cate.

A car instead of a metaphor.

She ordered it the next morning and arranged to pick it up the following afternoon. Meg offered to drive her to the dealership after school, so the kids could go. Kayla and Ben loved that idea.

"Hi, Dad, let's go for your car," said Ben as he ran through the front door and toward his dad, with Kayla on his heels. Lately, he'd stopped saying Daddy.

Jeff stretched out his arms with a smile. Cate hoped he understood about the car, that he was responding to more than the kids' enthusiasm.

"Is Dad gonna drive?" asked Kayla.

"When we get back to our neighborhood," said Cate.

"Hooray! I want to ride with Dad," said Ben.

Meg arrived with her two kids, and Cate, Jeff, and the kids piled into the car. "What kind of a car are you getting?" asked Evie.

"I don't know," said Jeff.

"A Toyota SUV, honey, like your old one."

"What color is it?" asked David.

"Silver?" said Jeff, looking at Cate.

"That was your old one. This one is navy blue." They reached the dealership, and Meg offered to follow them home.

"We'll be fine. Thanks for the taxi service."

"What taxi?" said Jeff.

"Mom means the ride from Meg," said Kayla.

The kids and Jeff looked at cars in the lot while Cate completed the paperwork, which took about an hour.

When they reached home, Cate and Jeff exchanged seats. With a foot on the brake, Jeff shifted into drive, released his foot, and allowed the car to inch forward. He braked, and the car jerked to a stop. "Gently, honey." Cate looked at the kids and frowned. "You guys go into the house. I'll come get you in a little while."

"No," said Ben. "I want to ride with Dad."

"He drives your car," said Kayla.

"I'll be careful," said Jeff. With trepidation, she let the kids remain.

Outside the cul-de-sac was a circle with houses on both sides before a straight road connected the circle to the main street. Jeff drove around the circle as Cate watched carefully for children; he eased into the driveway, stopped, and reached for the garage door opener.

"We haven't set it for this car, but you've got the right idea." Cate checked to make sure Jeff had shifted to park and nodded to Kayla, who used the garage door keypad. The door opened, and the space for Jeff's car yawned. Slowly, he maneuvered the car into place and sat, examining the controls and the interior.

"I used to drive this car."

"One just like it," said Cate.

"It's good," he said, with a hint of satisfaction. Then he exited the car, walked into the house, and closed the door, with Cate a few steps behind him. She knocked on the door, and Jeff opened it.

"You forgot me, honey."

"Oh, sorry." Cate's eyes filled with tears. Jeff looked at her, confused.

"I wish you understood, honey. I wish you could cry with me." But Cate knew she'd have to cry alone.

* * *

Just before dinner, Meg called to see how it went with the car.

"What drives me nuts is his inconsistency," said Cate. "He pilots the car into the garage, then he shuts the door and leaves me there." Cate carried the cell phone back to her home office. "At least they haven't given up on him in rehab. It's damn close to a year, and we can expect precious little improvement in the second year."

"Can you detect change when you work with him at home?"

"Glacial, more from week to week. The kids miss their old dad, but their lives go on. They've adapted better than I have."

"They're kids. The burden is on you."

"Thank heavens for family and friends."

"Does that include Jack?"

"He's a friend. A special friend."

"I came across a word that's perfect for you. *Coddiwomple.* It's English slang."

"What does it mean?"

"To travel with purpose toward a vague destination."

"That's what I'm doing, all right."

"Yes, in all the corners of your life."

"All the corners?"

"That's what I said." They ended the call, with Cate reflecting.

CHAPTER FORTY-SIX:

Late September

Cate and Jeff perched on the edge of a well-used couch, lumpy and chocolate brown, meeting with Jeff's treatment team. Dr. Janiscek's huge desk, piled high with journals and books, reminded Cate of her office at the university, but the setting anchored Cate in a different reality.

The team discussed Jeff's overall progress, what they observed, and what recent neuropsychological testing confirmed. They reviewed Jeff's treatment goals.

"How long will Cognitive OT continue?" asked Cate.

"As long as Jeff benefits. He's still learning skills that help him cope, so we're not close to discharge," said Lori.

"Cate, how are you doing?" asked Dr. Janiscek.

"My friend Meg asked me that yesterday." Cate's eyes moistened. "I said, *Je suis désolée.*"

"Desolated?" asked Dr. Janiscek. "In French, that's an apology. Are you apologizing?"

"Maybe." Cate thought of the night before the accident, the next morning, and Jack. "Jeff and I were working some things out when the accident happened. What I regret is my contribution to our problems."

"Tension you can't resolve makes everything harder," said Dr. Hunter, the psychologist. "You haven't mentioned that to me, but you're welcome to talk about it."

"I'll try to talk more about our relationship." But not about Jack, thought Cate, as Jeff leaned toward her and touched the back of her hand.

"He senses your emotion, and that's a good sign," said Dr. Hunter. Cate turned her palm upward, squeezed Jeff's hand, and managed a subdued smile.

"I love you, honey. You know I do, don't you?" said Cate.

"Yes," he said. "I do."

"Cate, you look dejected," said Dr. Hunter.

"You help a lot, but I carry the sadness for both of us. There's so much he doesn't understand." She wiped away tears. "It's ten months, and there's less improvement in the second year."

"You're discouraged, but there's still hope, and there's still time," said Dr. Janiscek.

"Thanks, I'll try to let that in. We'll all try, won't we, Jeff?"

He gripped her hand.

"Any questions?" asked Dr. Janiscek.

"After this," said Emmie Rose, the social worker, "we're going to meet separately to talk about finances and insurance."

There were no questions for the rest of the team, and the meeting concluded.

* * *

On the way to the social work office, they stopped in the reception area for coffee. Jeff poured cups for Cate and Emmie Rose before pouring his.

"That's nice," said Emmie Rose. "Do you see that at home?"

"Not often," said Cate.

In her office, Emmie Rose asked how they were doing without Jeff's income. Cate glanced at Jeff, who hadn't a clue.

"I make a good salary as a university professor, which comes with family health insurance and other benefits," said Cate. In addition, there's Jeff's disability income, considerably less than the salary he took from his business, and reduced profits, which his partner generously shares. Cate planned to apply for Social Security benefits for Jeff in two months, when she could document a full year of disability.

"Good. Leaving aside medical expenses, what are your other costs?"

"At first, Jeff's long-term insurance covered help at home, but that stopped when he didn't need 24/7 supervision. We still have increased expenses for home care and extra help for the kids, what Jeff used to do."

"How about savings for the kids' college and your retirement?"

"We've put some money into college savings plans for the kids, but it won't be enough." Cate had reduced, for now, contributions to her retirement plans, but she and Jeff both had them. They had counted on Jeff's income. "I don't want to give up the house, but we have to make adjustments in how we live."

"Okay, let's talk about medical expenses." For the first year, health insurance had covered Jeff's medical care, but when Jeff exceeded the allotted number of visits allowed for Cognitive OT, they stopped paying. They continued to pay for neuropsych testing, Dr. Janiscek, and psychological care, although they argued about much of it.

Keith, their attorney, and Scott's partner had again told Cate not to worry about medical costs. He had, as promised, sent the hospital a letter guaranteeing payment once the claims process concluded. "Eventually," said Keith, "the other driver's insurance will pay to the limits of their coverage, and that will be enough for all of Jeff's medical expenses and part of his lost income. But they'll try to delay settlement or trial," he said, "hoping that your financial distress will force a smaller settlement. It's in your interest to wait until we know the degree of Jeff's permanent disability, the amount of his lost income, and the long-term costs of caring for him at home." When there was a settlement, some of that money would go to reimburse Jeff's health insurance company, a process called subrogation of benefits.

"We'll continue all the treatments we think are necessary," said Emmie Rose. "We know it takes several years to resolve an accident claim. If you think about it, the cost of unreimbursed care is an interest-free loan that we provide until settlement, a hidden healthcare cost that few consider."

"Thanks," said Cate. "We appreciate all the care and support that Sister Kenny provides. She looked at Jeff, who listened, and said nothing.

CHAPTER FORTY-SEVEN:

End of October

Cate and Jack had settled into a routine, a run once or twice a week followed by a shower, then tender or passionate lovemaking on his bed or on the couch in front of the large picture window, which felt daring, and once in the heat of August, upstairs in the open air on the terrace, followed by lunch at nearby places or delivered to Jack's apartment. Sometimes they worked for an hour in his place before or after lunch. Twice, they found a way to attend a concert together at Orchestra Hall.

They talked by cellphone at least once a day and exchanged texts throughout the day and on weekday evenings and weekends. Usually, Jack texted before he called to be sure she was free since Cate lived her life in two compartments.

Once, Jack forgot and called while Cate was reviewing homework with Kayla and Ben. "Hello," she said, and her chest hollowed when she heard Jack's voice. "I'll call you later." Her voice was stiff.

"Mom, are you okay?" asked Kayla. "You sounded nervous."

"It was about work," said Cate, and she forced her attention back to the kids.

Later that evening, Jack apologized.

"Thanks, but that wasn't okay. I never want to choose between you and the kids, even for a phone call. It pulls me apart."

Another mishap occurred the same week. Cate sat on a chair in the bedroom, talking with Jack about their day, while Jeff watched a TV show downstairs. Earlier than expected, Jeff returned to the bedroom. Cate hurried off the phone, feeling unnerved and disloyal to both.

She arranged a meeting with Meg, in Meg's office, to discuss these misadventures. "I do okay when I keep things separate, and it's worth the effort." She thought about her office, the pictures on her wall and bookshelves, the executive chair, and the way, before the accident, all the parts of her life flowed together. "But sometimes it drives me nuts. If I ever had to choose between Jack and the kids, the choice would be easy. But sometimes I think about what I might do if the kids were older, out of the house. Would I leave Jeff?"

"Would you?"

"Life with Jack would be pleasant and easy, and Jeff has lost his zest, so it's possible to contemplate life without him. Then I remember those marriage vows—for better or for worse, 'til death do us part—and know I'd never abandon him. I still love him, at least the idea of him, the idea of marriage. At times, it's only obligation."

"What about life without Jack?"

"I couldn't bear it. I couldn't survive. At least not now."

"Then it's clear. You're less stressed with Jack than you'd be without him."

"Jeff and the kids don't know about Jack. It's a lie by omission. But the other day, Jack called when I was with the kids, and I lied directly."

"It's complicated."

"It feels crazy. I can manage a lie of omission but not a direct lie."

"It's a thin distinction, but a real one, at least to me. Cate, you're caring for Jeff as well as anyone could possibly do. You're meeting the kids' needs. And you're managing a busy career. You couldn't do any of it if you ignored your emotional needs."

That's true." Cate sighed. "But it sounds like bullshit rationalization."

"I'd call it a compromise. You're honest with Jack, with me, and with yourself. That's as honest as the situation allows, if you're to keep functioning."

Cate sighed. "It's an impossible situation. Sometimes in the middle of the night, I feel stuck in mire."

"If the sludge gets too thick, call me. Right now, you look clean and dry, so hug your enabler."

"My enabler?" Cate couldn't resist a smile and a hug. "You're my oldest friend. My BFF."

"And you're mine."

They left Meg's office and walked along the river, where autumn colored the trees along the banks.

* * *

Cate and Jack knew it would be harder, less discreet when it got too cold to run outside. They would have to run in the University Fieldhouse and travel to Jack's apartment from there, but they wanted to make it work.

Cate liked that Jack talked to her about his family. Harvard had recently promoted Jack's older son, still single but living with his girlfriend of several years, to associate professor of history. Will, his son on the faculty of the NYU medical school, expected a boy, and Jack was excited about his first grandchild.

"Liz would've loved that grandchild, and I would've loved to share that experience with her," said Jack. "Not having grandchildren made it hard for her to let go, even at the end."

"You miss Liz a lot, don't you?"

"I shouldn't talk so much about her."

"Of course you should. You're talking about what's important to you. Don't ever stop." Cate leaned forward, attentive.

Jack often asked about Jeff and his progress, about the children, about her, and his interest and concern for Jeff felt genuine and compassionate. Jack understood the pain of lost intimacy, the way Jeff's TBI robbed him of agency. He accepted the complexity of Cate's marriage. Cate talked to Jack about Sally, what it had felt like to lose her sister at twelve, and how Jeff's injury brought that pain to the surface. Jack never failed to listen well.

Early in the summer, a year and a half after Liz passed, Jack decided to redecorate the apartment and make it his. Cate looked with him at paint and fabric samples, at furniture, and teased him about his bachelor pad. By early October, the renovation was complete. The new style was minimalist, the colors warm and comforting, free of hunter green and burgundy, damask, dated prints, and heavy furnishings. In the new kitchen, stainless steel appliances, light oak floors and cabinetry, and granite counters, golden brown and swirled with gray and ivory, displaced every trace of white. Elsewhere, slate gray leather couches and chairs with modern lines, parchment walls, and light gray carpeting blended well with artifacts collected from around the world.

Pictures of Liz, Jack, and their children rested on tansu chests and on Jack's beloved antique Japanese coffee table, a large rectangle of Zenkova elm with black lacquered legs, which often held their lunch.

Jack loved his new space, and Cate felt comfortable there. She thought of it as Jack's place, with bits of her.

"We've been together for four months. Tell me what it's like for you," said Jack.

"It feels like separate lives and separate spaces. Part dream and part nightmare, except for the kids. Not all nightmare, I guess, because I still love Jeff. The last thing I want is to hurt him. Or the kids."

"That's important to you, and I'm always glad to hear it."

"I tell myself that I wouldn't be much good to Jeff and the kids if I felt emotionally dead. You help me stay alive."

"You're alive. You're present in this apartment. With me."

"I'm also present in my prosaic suburban house, with its large backyard and the garden that I tended all summer, planting and weeding with the kids, sometimes with Jeff. I also have memories, twelve years of them."

"That describes the separate spaces."

"But you're right, there's only me, wherever I am. It takes constant effort to keep my head on straight."

"It's a lot less risky for me."

"What do you get out of this? I know, but I need to hear it."

"Until you came along, I was pickled and sitting on a shelf."

Cate laughed and at once felt lighter. "That is a good visual, although it would take a large jar to hold you and you'd have to be on the floor, not a shelf. You are salty."

"You're pretty spicy yourself."

"See. That's why it works."

They opened a bottle of wine, spread some gruyère on crackers, and teased each other for another hour.

CHAPTER FORTY-EIGHT:

December 2013

After a full year of recovery, Jeff worked for an hour twice each week in his lab. He'd improved enough to drive alone on the highway during daylight hours when traffic remained light if roads were clear and snow-free. Initially, Bill reported that Jeff sat at the desk and stared. He didn't work with embryos; he didn't talk on the phone with client farmers. But eventually, he began to ask questions like, "Where are you sending them?" as Bill packed embryos in dry ice.

After talking to Bill, Cate accompanied Jeff to work for a couple of hours and took detailed notes and pictures. Then she led Jeff through several dry runs at home.

One Thursday, she and Bill watched as Jeff put on gloves, packed dry ice in plastic, and placed it in a cardboard box, pausing each step to check the notes crammed onto a single logbook page. "You can do it. We rehearsed this at home," said Cate when Jeff faltered.

"Nice job," said Bill. "Please be very careful with the embryos."

"Maybe you should prepare another box first," said Cate.

Bill agreed. Jeff checked the logbook and repeated the steps.

Then, following Cate's prompts and the logbook, he removed an embryo from the freezer, protected it with Styrofoam, added it to the box, added more dry ice, and sealed the box. He filled the second box with another embryo.

"What's the next step?" asked Cate. He glanced at the logbook.

"FedEx."

"How will they know where to send it?" asked Cate. Referring to the logbook again, Jeff signed into the FedEx account, printed labels, and copied addresses from Bill's notes.

"Good," said Bill. "I think you get it, but it's best for me or someone else in the lab to check your work, at least for now."

"Do you think Jeff can start talking to farmers?" asked Cate.

"He's not ready," said Bill. "I overheard him tell a farmer that he was fine and back to work, and I had to tell that guy about Jeff's injury and lack of insight."

"I could do the same thing—watch you, make notes and pictures for Jeff to practice talking to farmers at home."

"A conversation is more complicated than packing embryos," said Bill, "but let me think about it."

Jeff packed a third embryo into a box, addressed a label, and completed the online FedEx transaction to arrange pickup before he left with Cate.

On the drive home, Jeff watched the road, turned at the right places, and responded to traffic and to traffic signals. He could drive in safe conditions. Follow rules. Use judgment when the kinds of decisions he might need to make were clear, circumscribed, and possible to anticipate. "Honey, I'll bet there are conversations with farmers that you *could* have. It's kind of like driving. Work out the rules and the kinds of judgments you might have to make, practice them, and figure out what you have to anticipate." Cate decided to call Bill and try to understand the process of talking to farmers and what issues might arise. Maybe Lori could help.

Cate could tell that the idea pleased Jeff. Despite his blunted emotion, she could discern a modicum of pleasure.

The kids, especially Kayla, had learned to read Jeff too. Last evening, Ben had said, "I can tell when you're gonna talk to us, Dad." Jeff looked up. "When you're not slumped up, like a ball."

"Yeah, when you feel good, you sit up and look around," said Kayla. "Sometimes, if we talk to you, we can get you to sit up."

"Like now," said Ben. "You were slumped up, but now you're not. You look tired, but I can tell you're happy."

"Even if you don't smile," said Kayla.

Sometimes Jeff began interactions with the kids. Usually not. In general, Cate and the kids exerted energy, and Jeff absorbed it, responding with constrained vitality.

Jeff had learned to use Cognitive OT skills to anticipate and plan for evenings, gatherings, outings, and work. He'd begun to run again, alone or with Scott, in the neighborhood when sidewalks were not slippery, or at the fitness club, where he lifted weights with a trainer and began to rebuild muscle. He looked good physically—normal—but that proved to be a double-edged sword. People engaged him and expected a normal response.

Cate and Jeff had sex the few times that Cate initiated it, which Cate continued because it felt important to maintain that bond—although, for the most part, it was a mechanical act that left Cate hungry for emotional heat.

One Sunday morning in the last half of December, Jeff surprised her when he touched her shoulder and then her breast, gently, the way he used to caress her, and wrapped his arms around her with subdued playfulness. "I love you," he said for the first time since the accident, with a kiss that began with a touch of his lips and grew. Cate watched her mouth respond. It felt like she was watching a different couple. Hardening of her nipples and familiar tingling pulled her into the moment. She kissed him, exploring his tongue with hers, and he kissed her breasts and tickled her nipples with his tongue. They touched and kissed until she was making love with eagerness. They lay facing each other, eyes open at first, touching, then closed as their hips began to move, both moaning softly until he released, but he continued until she throbbed with a prolonged climax that awakened in her more than physicality. It felt intimate.

Afterward, as Cate lay on her back, Jeff beside her with his eyes closed, she reflected on the past few weeks, certain that something had changed. At this point, any discernable improvement occurred from month to month. Jeff had begun to bring a spark to family interactions, a glow that unsettled the balance she'd achieved. How could she love two men and sustain a divided life? The relationship with Jack, its frankness and openness, and perhaps her work, the part that didn't involve Jack, had felt like the most honest part of her existence. In order to survive, she'd deceived Jeff and her children.

Now that a year had passed since the accident, with minimal recovery expected in the second year, perhaps the team at Sister Kenny could forecast the endpoint of Jeff's recovery. If only Cate could see the journey's end, she could decide—objectively, rationally—what kind of life she wanted to lead, how she might satisfy her own emotional needs and care for her family. She would call Dr. Janiscek's office first thing tomorrow to arrange a meeting.

It was nine o'clock Sunday morning. Beside her, Jeff had fallen asleep. She could hear the children downstairs and hoped they'd been sufficiently quiet. She closed her eyes and, after several minutes, fell into a brief and restless sleep.

An hour later, the screech of tires, the crunch of metal grinding against metal, the sound of shattering glass, and the wail of sirens jolted Cate to wakefulness, her face and pajamas drenched with sweat. She sat on the edge of the bed, breathing rapidly, calming herself, until her heart slowed, and she had fully awakened from the nightmare. Jeff was no longer in bed, and she could hear noises and voices downstairs. She tossed her damp pajamas into the laundry, rubbed a wet washcloth over her body without showering, dried herself, threw on jeans and a sweatshirt, and hurried downstairs, feeling an urge, almost irresistible, to review medical records and police reports from the day of the accident that she had collected but had not until now wanted to read.

"I helped Dad make pancakes," said Kayla.

Hiding her distress, Cate greeted her family as pleasantly as possible. "They smell delicious. I'll have some in a little while, after I do a little work in my office." Cate headed down the hall, glad that her home office was isolated from the rest of the house.

As if reliving the accident could help, Cate pulled from her closet the box of medical records and police reports, including the accident reconstruction compiled by state troopers. On top lay a police photo of the Dodge Challenger, the car that caused the accident, lying on its side. Below it lay pictures of Jeff's SUV turned sideways on the shoulder with the windshield shattered and blood-tinged, the driver's compartment collapsed, the steering wheel pressed so closely against the seat that it looked like there had been no room left for Jeff. Witnesses had described Jeff as barely conscious for five or ten minutes after the crash. First responders, who arrived shortly thereafter, described Jeff as minimally conscious in the front seat, which did not change during the fifteen minutes it took the emergency medical technicians to pry open Jeff's passenger door with the Jaws of Life and pull him from the crumpled vehicle; from the outset, because of the shattered windshield and altered consciousness, EMTs had assumed that Jeff had a traumatic brain injury and radioed ahead to the HCMC emergency room, telling them what to expect.

Cate flipped to the emergency room records and found herself in the stabilization room, overwhelmed, trying to make sense of desperate attention focused on Jeff.

She pushed back her chair and paced until the apparition cleared. Then she read and reread the notes of Dr. O'Reilly, the emergency room physician, and Dr. Watkins, the neurosurgeon, including the operating room report, all of which described Jeff's injuries in terms both clinical and stark.

Although Cate had reviewed a small portion of what the box contained, she could absorb no more. Only the police report and accident reconstruction added new content to her understanding; the rest crystallized memory. She'd return to it in the future, she knew, but for now, the box belonged on the closet shelf behind the closed closet door. She leaned her back against that door and pressed.

Back in the kitchen, Kayla had helped Jeff make a fresh batch of pancakes, and Cate ate, tentatively at first, but the familiar taste and family chatter soothed her. "Hey, these are delicious. Thanks for making them," said Cate. She had a second cup of coffee as Kayla rinsed the dishes and silverware and put them in the dishwasher.

Cate, wanting to get away from the house, suggested a ride to the Ridgedale mall to finish Christmas shopping and the kids raced to the car. Jeff surprised her by climbing into the driver's seat of the SUV. Before Christmas, the parking lot would be crowded, difficult to negotiate, but Cate willed her thumping heart to still and let him drive. She watched every move as he started the car, pressed the accelerator, backed into the turnaround, and steered into the street—suppressing, with limited success, images of the damaged vehicles hidden in the box inside her closet. As Jeff drove slowly and carefully, negotiating the busy parking lot with sudden obstacles and close calls, Cate monitored every element of his performance. She felt relief when the drive, which seemed like a video game, ended, and they entered the store. They completed the shopping easily. When they once again reached the car, Cate aimed for the driver's seat and, to her relief, Jeff crawled into the passenger's seat. She checked everyone's seatbelts and headed home.

CHAPTER FORTY-NINE:

January 2014

Cate's review of Jeff's medical records and police reports reminded her of the discussion she had with Dr. Boulder one year ago. She remembered the life-size model of a skull and brain, sitting like a driver in the seat of a model car, how the brain crashed against the front of the skull and rebounded, coup and contrecoup, and how the bottom of the brain rubbed like a washboard against the uneven floor of the skull.

As she sat alone on Dr. Janiscek's couch, lumpy and brown, remembering, she wanted the best estimate of what Jeff would be like in another year, when his brain stopped healing.

"It's not like a switch is flipped," said Dr. Janiscek, gently. "A healed brain can still learn."

"I'm looking for answers, not inspiration. From the testing, from what you see. I asked Dr. Boulder the same question a year ago, and she gave me a vague answer. When I pushed, she guessed that in a year—that's now—Jeff might be able to do limited work with instructions from others, with limited problem-solving skills. That turned out to be right, although I hoped he'd have more abilities than he does."

"What did she say about his personality, when you pushed?"

"There was a chance that lack of interest in doing things, his lack of passion and social awareness, would disable him the most."

"What do you think about her predictions?"

"Pretty accurate. At times there's a trace of his old warmth, but he's not the same."

"She was brave to guess, and that's partly what it was. Now it's a year later, and we know a lot more, but it's still true that every TBI is different, that every brain heals in a different way, even in the second year. If I had to guess, though, I'd expect only modest improvement in Jeff's executive functions—planning, making decisions, following through—and the same with warm-heartedness and passion. I can't predict exactly what that will look and feel like."

"I want your best estimate."

"He'll be minimally better, with the same issues."

"I was afraid of that."

"We still have a year to go, and I've been pleasantly surprised before."

"Pleasantly surprised. That's what Dr. Boulder said."

"Of course. For one thing, it's possible. For another, it's the language of hope."

Cate sat for a long time in her car, reflecting, trying to predict the unpredictable, what interacting with Jeff would look and feel like. Then she drove to the university and sat at her worktable, staring at the wine-red chair.

CHAPTER FIFTY:

Late January

The ice arena at the Hopkins Pavilion was cold, but the adults, bundled in winter coats, didn't mind. The Zamboni had completed a run, and the children skated on resurfaced ice, hockey sticks in hand. Kayla and Evie worked with the girls on puck-passing skills at one end of the ice, and at the other end, Ben, David, and other boys did short and quick shifts, learning how to position arms and sticks as they turned.

"How's Ben doing?" asked Meg.

"Better." He'd had a setback, throwing up every morning, unable to make decisions. Cate had taken him to see June a few times. He'd realized that his father wasn't going to improve any further and had grown anxious. "All those behaviors stopped, and he seems back to normal." Jeff, focused on the ice, seemed to ignore this discussion.

"That's a relief," said Meg.

"Look at the four of them. They're getting good," said Scott.

"Yeah," said Jeff.

"Makes me want to get on the ice," said Scott. "Haven't played hockey since college."

"I know you were captain of your high school team. Didn't know you played in college," said Cate.

"Just pickup games. I wasn't good enough to make the team at the U of M, unlike Jeff, who played for Harvard. Hey, Jeff, let's rent some skates when the ice is free, and we can show the kids how it's done." The pavilion didn't rent skates, but a local business had taken space inside the pavilion as an experiment and had equipment that fit adults.

"Not a good idea," said Meg with a frown and a vigorous shake of her head.

"No way," said Cate. "Not even with a helmet." There was already an increased risk of Alzheimer's-like cognitive loss occurring many years after a TBI, added to existing impairment. Another injury could devastate. At least his attention had improved. Several months ago, Dr. Boulder had started Jeff on modafinil to improve attention, and donepezil, a medication first used in Alzheimer's, and also used to improve cognition in brain-injured patients.

"Helmets come with the skates," said Scott. Jeff stood and shifted his weight quickly from foot to foot several times, then stood on each leg for several seconds. "Look, he's practicing his balance. It might be good for him to try."

"He's balancing on shoes, not skates," said Cate, torn between Jeff's display of enthusiasm and his safety. "A concussion could do a lot of damage."

"We'll skate slowly, and I'll be right there with him," said Scott.

"I want to skate," said Jeff.

"If you try, will you promise to be careful?" asked Cate.

"Yes," said Jeff.

"Scott, you'd better be *very* careful," said Meg.

"He'll be fine," said Scott. "We'll rent skates and helmets as soon as the kids finish practice."

The four adults settled into their seats. Ben did a quick skate toward the bleachers and waved. "Stay with the exercise," yelled the coach. "You have to keep your head in what you're doing," but he looked at the parents and gave a quick thumbs up, drawing smiles.

Across the ice, Kayla and Evie worked on one-footed hops, edge control, and snowplow stops.

"Stopping looks like the hardest part," said Cate.

"It can be," said Meg, who had figure skated as a child. "It's body control and balance, pretty much like gymnastics. You have to put your weight on the front of the skate, or you land on your butt."

"It's not the butt I'm worried about."

A whistle blew, and the kids cleared the ice.

"Okay, Jeff. We're on," said Scott. Outside the enclosed ice arena, the dads donned skates and helmets. As soon as the Zamboni finished its work, they stepped through the door onto the ice. The moms and kids zipped up coats and put on gloves or mittens to stay warm in the bleachers.

It took the men a few minutes to look reasonably steady. Jeff held onto the wall until he seemed comfortable, then held onto Scott and worked to improve his balance. To Cate's relief, body memories returned quickly, and Jeff began to glide slowly along the ice, showing more confidence as minutes passed. They skated around the perimeter, Scott close enough to break Jeff's fall, if needed.

"Go, Dad," yelled Kayla.

All four kids cheered. Scott stopped to support Jeff as they both bowed before continuing the circuit. Halfway around, they began to skate a little faster. A smile crept across Jeff's face. When the dads reached their families, they stopped once more and bowed. This time, Jeff stood alone, not hanging onto Scott.

"Want to join us?" asked Scott.

"Not on rentals," said Meg, the former figure skater. "I'll bring my own skates next time."

"We can all bring our own," said Cate.

"Nice. I'd love to see you and Jeff skate together," said Scott. He tapped Jeff's back, and they skated to the center of the arena, away from the railing.

CHAPTER FIFTY-ONE:

March

Cate and Jack sat on Jack's slate couch surrounded by soothing parchment walls. On one of the antique tansu chests, a snapshot of Cate and Jack at a faculty gathering, innocent enough to anyone but the two of them, had joined the photos of Liz and Jack's family.

Jack had loved Meg's word. "That's what it is," said Jack, "a *coddiwomple,* this journey we're all taking. A mix of comfort and excitement."

Since winter, they'd run at the Fieldhouse at least once a week and driven afterward to Jack's condo. Now that it was spring, Cate drove to Jack's apartment, and they ran outside, along the river. The routine worked, and Cate felt less exposed than she had anticipated, although Jennifer had figured out their relationship. Thankfully, Jennifer remained discreet.

Cate turned to look through the picture window behind her at the vista that stretched northeast, the site of many enjoyable runs. When she looked at Jack again, her eyes were moist. "You do know that I love you, don't you?"

"Of course, and I love you." His brow furrowed. "It's strange in a way. I couldn't grieve for Liz until we got together."

"Grief is part of love, so it's not so strange that one love frees another. Remember, you were the one who compared your loss and mine. You said yours was finite and distinct, mine continuous and evolving, but even yours evolved." She paused to wipe her eyes. "The problem is, mine is still evolving, and it gets harder for me as Jeff improves. This divided life."

"It sounds like something has changed?"

"It feels like Jeff is more of a person, although he'll never regain everything, and he probably won't work, at least not with the same effectiveness."

"I'm glad he's getting better, at least a little."

"I haven't wanted to say this to you, but Jeff and I made love a few times because I thought we should." She looked away, then back.

"I'm not surprised. I've known you have to live your life, all of it."

"It doesn't feel satisfying or intimate like it does with you."

"Intimacy. Will that improve with time? With Jeff?"

"I thought so once, but I've learned that it's not possible for him. He doesn't initiate, and I won't either, ever again."

"This is a hard subject, but I love the honesty between us," said Jack. Their eyes met, and neither faltered. "Something's bugging you. What is it?"

"I think it's the deception. It's always bothered me that I'm not being honest with Jeff or with the kids. Especially the kids."

"Has something about that changed too?"

"I have a lot more time to think now that I'm less overwhelmed, less desperate. More time to feel the loss the kids and I have suffered, the division in my life. Time adds perspective."

"And perspective adds guilt?"

"That too."

"I think you can cut yourself some slack. I do. What you experienced with Jeff's accident would devastate anyone, and you've shown remarkable strength. You've kept your family intact and done everything possible to give Jeff the best life possible."

"Except faithfulness."

"You needed intimacy to survive. You still do, and I need it too. I think about those nights alone in Japan, my last sabbatical, without

Liz. Pretending. Not grieving. I didn't realize how lonely I was until our relationship changed."

"That's another thing. I worry that our relationship is holding you back. It's almost like I have two families, and you have half of one."

"That's the Cate I know. Kind and considerate. Look, I don't have the burden of a divided life. It makes sense to be discreet at work, but my kids do know about us. It's not holding me back, and if it ever does, I'll talk about it. I can make that decision for myself."

"That helps." Cate laughed. "Who knew collaboration could be so complex?"

"It works. It's our part of the *coddiwomple*."

"We can never marry. I won't leave Jeff."

"I wouldn't like you if you did. You wouldn't be the person I respect."

"Jeff needs me, and the children need our family."

"And you?"

"I need our family too."

"Cate, I admire you. Despite everything, you've persevered. You've tried to make sure that life remains an adventure for Kayla and Ben, and that your life has purpose."

"Yeah. That's an important part of the *coddiwomple*."

"Yes, it is," said Jack. He reached for Cate's hand, and she took it. His hand felt warm and reassuring. A hand but not a crutch. Cate stared out the picture window. She thought about the routes she and Jack had run, the endless variety of paths and options, over bridges, across islands, and back to security or its illusion. Her eyes rested on the river.

"I think it works for now," said Cate. "But I can't help wondering when and if this ends for us."

"It ends when and if it wants to, on its own terms, and I'm not saying it should," said Jack. "I do know that it would end with respect, not with anger or hatred because that's never been part of it for us." Jack rested an arm on her shoulder and grinned. "We would still collaborate."

"Even without our *coddiwomple*?"

"Coddiwomples evolve."

"I had a dream the other night. You and I were standing on the Stone Arch Bridge, watching the Mississippi, and a drop with Jeff's face floated past. I was swimming alongside Jeff, but I also stood on the bridge with you. Divided and somehow whole. I had to be there every ninety days to watch another drop of Jeff float by, and I knew I would be there, no matter what. Standing with you on the bridge, swimming with Jeff."

"Nice dream," said Jack.

"But it's a dream. Dreams always end."

"Yours doesn't end. You keep swimming, and the drops keep flowing."

"Yes, they do. Like the river."

A NOTE ABOUT JEFF AND CATE

There are a vast number of stories one might tell about people and families who cope with traumatic brain injury (TBI). This is true because TBI has many causes, degrees of severity, specific symptoms, degrees of recovery, and outcomes.

This novel tells the story of one person with TBI and his family, chosen to show how the loss of warmth, drive, creativity, and insight affects Jeff, Cate, and their children. There are no statistics to show how many people have stories like this one, but I have seen several variations of this kind of recovery, and many other patterns of injury and recovery over the years. Although we know a lot about TBI, we still know far too little about this common tragedy.

TBI: AN OVERVIEW

Falls cause nearly half of TBI injuries. Other common causes are motor vehicle crashes and assaults, followed by bike accidents and child abuse. Sports injuries, often in the news, cause TBI, and war injuries are another important cause. The elderly (from falls) and the homeless (from falls and trauma) are at high risk.

TBIs are divided into mild (includes concussion), moderate, and severe. Most are mild and nearly all recover completely from single injuries. The impact of multiple sports concussions remains a focus of research, as does the impact of blast injuries and multiple TBIs for soldiers. TBIs are also divided into closed—a bump, blow, or jolt to the head—and open—a penetrating injury such as a gunshot.

The number of people who suffer from TBI is at best a rough estimate. Many individuals with mild TBI do not seek care; some do not consult physicians or go to emergency rooms, so their TBI remains undiagnosed. The important story about sports injuries in professional athletes and children continues to evolve, including the issue of Chronic Traumatic Encephalopathy in professional athletes. And much research continues so that we can better understand the impact of TBI on soldiers, including blast injuries; TBI is considered the signature injury of the Iraq and Afghanistan wars.

Persistent symptoms of moderate to severe TBI include cognitive and personality issues

- *Cognitive changes*, which may be prominent or subtle, affect attention, concentration, memory, speed of information processing, and higher executive functions (think of what an executive does—he/she attends to complex issues, shifts attention from one problem to another, focuses on several tasks at once, manipulates concepts in memory, and uses judgment to make and implement decisions).
- *Personality changes* may include apathy (lack of drive and initiative); lack of insight and awareness of their own TBI symptoms; aggression or behavioral outbursts; disturbances of mood such as depression, anxiety, and irritability; and paranoia.

There are important time periods when recovery can be assessed for moderate to severe TBI:

- Much improvement occurs in the first few weeks. Improvement continues at a steadily declining rate, and three, six, and twelve months are useful times to assess recovery. Brain healing is often considered complete at two years.
- Yet people may still improve real world function by learning compensatory strategies after two years, which suggests that new neural pathways can develop thereafter.

Statistical estimates from Centers for Disease Control (CDC):

- 2.5 million TBI patients visit ERs each year in the United States; 85% have mild TBI.
- 5.3 million men, women, and children live with TBI-related disability in the United States today.
- 223,000 TBI-related hospitalizations occurred in 2019.
- 176 Americans died from TBI-related injuries each day in 2020.
- 15% of U.S. high-school students self-reported one or more sports or recreation-related concussions within the preceding twelve months; almost all recover—but the number of students with chronic issues remains unknown
- TBI costs for individuals, families, and society with permanent

injuries are great. In the United States, Americans spend $37.8 billion each year on TBI care. Average lifetime treatment costs are $600 thousand to $1.9 million per individual, not considering mental health costs for affected individuals and families, and not considering other lifetime costs for that are economically important, i.e., $69 billion for work loss, and $137 billion for lost quality of life. Many who suffer from TBI have mounting medical bills and become, or are, indigent.

In addition, perhaps 600,000 people—or more— have TBI from war injuries*

*From 2000 through the first quarter of 2013, some estimate that 2.4 million soldiers were discharged from service. If one assumes that 25% of these soldiers have TBI, the total number affected would be 600,000. While far from trivial, war injuries contribute far fewer individuals to the social burden of TBI disability than do falls, motor vehicle crashes, assaults, sports injuries, and other causes of TBI. War injuries are often complicated by Posttraumatic Stress Disorder (PTSD), and Major Depressive Disorder.

FURTHER READING

1. *In An Instant*, Lee and Bob Woodruff, Random House, 2008. The story of a TV news anchorman, who sustains a traumatic brain injury covering the Iraq war, and how his long recovery affected him and his family
2. *Mindstorms*, the complete guide for families living with traumatic brain injury, Lee Woodruff and John W. Cassidy, Da Capo Press, 2009. Although dated, this book has much useful information for contemporary readers
3. *A Stitch in Time*, Lauren Marks, Simon and Schuster, 2017. A memoir by a woman who had a ruptured arterial brain aneurysm that caused a hemorrhagic stroke, a kind of acquired brain injury—not a traumatic brain injury—which affected mainly language abilities
4. *Textbook of Traumatic Brain Injury*, Third Edition, Edited by Jonathan M. Silver, M.D., Thomas W. McAllister, M.D., .and David B. Arciniegas, M.D., American Psychiatric Publishing, 2019. The definitive textbook about traumatic brain injury, occasionally reissued with updated information
5. Google CDC traumatic brain injury for updated information

Brain Injury Association of America, http://biausa.org has many useful links, including some helpful in finding care near you.

Minnesota Brain Injury Alliance, http://www.braininjurymn.org, is a consumer-oriented organization founded by families and providers, full of useful and practical information, including how to understand brain injury (as this book went to press, it's under Resource Facilitation>Library Articles>Understanding Traumatic Brain Injury (Parts 1-4)

ACKNOWLEDGEMENTS

Many people guided and informed me in the process of writing *Accidental Journey*. Without Minnesota Book Award winner Peter Geye, leader of the one-year Novel Writing Project for advanced students at the Loft Literary Center in Minneapolis, your reading lamp would not have found this novel. Others in my cohort of twelve writers in the NWP, especially Brian Duren and Cary Griffith, offered helpful criticism throughout the year and thereafter, and Peter Geye helped with two subsequent manuscript consultations. Other teachers at the Loft introduced me to the elements of fiction writing and helped me begin the essential journey from technical journal writing to fiction. I took my first three courses with Kate St. Vincent Vogl, and she provided a rich introduction to the elements of fiction in her warm and respectful classroom. Other important Loft teachers were Kevin Fenton, Deborah Fries, David Housewright, Brian Malloy, and Allison Wyss. In one of these classes, I met Jim Kaufmann, who provided useful review and commentary, and with whom I still meet monthly for friendly conversation. I also meet regularly with Brian Duren and Cary Griffith.

In working with people who have traumatic brain injury and their families over the years, I have had the pleasure of collaborating with many at Courage Kenny, including physical medicine doctor Jennine Speier, neuropsychologists Kyle Harvison and George Montgomery, occupational therapists specializing in cognitive rehabilitation Sue Newman and Joette Zola, and psychologist David Lund. Sue, Joette, Kyle, David, and Jennine provided specific help that informed my novel.

Elinor Hands, one of the founders of the Brain Injury Alliance, and its Chief Executive Officer, David King, provided important critiques. Neuropsychiatrist John W. Cassidy, founder of the TBI program at McLean Hospital in Boston and Chief Medical Officer & CEO of Nexus Health Systems in Houston, reviewed the novel for accuracy and coherence and made many helpful suggestions. At Hennepin County Medical Center, neurosurgery nurse practitioner Carla Cerra described the acute ICU care of brain injured patients with thoughtfulness and concern, and emergency medicine physician Brian Mahoney, along with the skilled emergency room nurses, let me shadow them in the stabilization room, where evaluation and acute care are remarkable. I have also collaborated over the years with neuropsychologists Michael Fuhrman and Gary Krupp, and with neurologists Teresa Tran-Lim and other, and have learned much from them.

In writing about Cate, understanding her as a woman, my wife, Joanie, provided essential guidance and perspective. David Duxbury taught me much about veterinary science and how characters like Jeff improve the quality of milk. My colleague, Kim Fitch, and her son, Gavin, and husband, Chris, provided lots of information about Quarter Midget racing and a couple of delightful days at the racing track in Elko New Market, Minnesota. Chris Lautenschlager of the Marcy-Holmes Neighborhood Association and Kristen Eide-Tollefson of Dinkytown's Book House, and keeper of the Dinkytown archives, shepherded me through Dinkytown's history and lore. I had a delightful correspondence with composer Elizabeth Raum about her piece, *Four Elements for Violin and Trombone***.** Attorney Robin Landy helped me understand the legal and financial obstacles that TBI patients and their families face, as did the social workers at Courage Kenny. The anecdote about Flaubert was inspired by a New Yorker article written by John Lahr about Julianne Moore, that uses the idea, regular and orderly in life, violent and original in work.

Thanks to the members of my first writing group, June Blumenson, Judy Liautaud, and Pamm Smith. And to the members of my group with a common interest in writing and psychoanalysis, especially Leslie Morris and Madelon Sprengnether. I owe much to the members of the Narrative Medicine Collaborative at the Institute of Advanced Study, University of Minnesota, including Jennifer Gunn, Gloria Levin, MJ Maynes, Leslie Morris, EmmaLee Pallai, Larry Savett, Madelon Sprengnether, and others. I benefitted from other writing groups that include Hal Steiger, some of the same people, and others. Many of the people mentioned above have read part or all of the novel, and to them I am grateful. Readers also include my wife, Joanie, my sons, Daniel and Andrew, Elinor Hands, David King, Polly McCormack, Jennine Speier, and Michael Trangle. I hope I have mentioned everyone; if not, I apologize.

For all of the elements in this novel, from fiction to the intricate aspects of traumatic brain injury care and description, any errors or omissions fall on my shoulders.

ABOUT THE AUTHOR

As a clinical and forensic psychiatrist and retired Adjunct Professor of Psychiatry at the University of Minnesota, Dr. Lentz has extensive experience with individuals and families who have coped with traumatic brain injury. He chose fiction as the best vehicle to make accessible this common, real, and poorly understood affliction—a story he is passionate to tell. He completed the Novel Writing Project at the Loft Literary Center in Minneapolis and is a participant in the Narrative Medicine Collaborative at the Institute of Advanced Study, University of Minnesota.

He graduated from the University of Rochester School of Medicine and Dentistry with an M.S in Neuropathology and an M.D. with Distinction in Research. Before turning to psychiatry, he studied pediatric nephrology at the University of Minnesota and served for two years as Chief of Pediatric Nephrology, Walter Reed Army Medical Center. He lives in downtown Minneapolis with his wife, a psychoanalyst in private practice. He enjoys spending time with family, including his two sons who live in the Twin Cities. Among his many interests, Richard serves on the board of the oldest community orchestra in Minneapolis.

Made in the USA
Monee, IL
20 March 2024